Arts Therapies and the Mental Health of Children and Young People

This second volume expands and develops the discussion on arts therapies begun in volume one on the field's relationship with children and young people's mental health, demonstrating further contemporary research within international contexts.

The book responds to a resounding call to address children and young people's mental health. It explores a unique mix of diverse arts modalities including art, music, dance, expressive arts, and drama, creating opportunities for discourse and discussion of how the different arts therapies cohere and relate to each other. Chapters are truly global in approach, ranging from schools in India to children's hospices in the United Kingdom, refugee transit camps in Greece, and residential care programmes for LGBTQ+ youth in the United States. Discussions from Greece and Taiwan, and innovative research from Israel, Norway, and Scotland are also featured with reference to diverse social, political, and cultural contexts. Ultimately, chapters prioritise the links between research, theory, and practice, providing accessible and implication-led dialogue on contemporary issues.

This book provides new insights into the expanding field of arts therapies and will be of great interest to arts therapists as well as academics and students in the fields of arts therapies, social work, psychotherapy, health psychology, and education.

Uwe Herrmann is a Professor on the MA Art Therapy programme, Weissensee University of Art Berlin, and Art Therapist, State Training Centre for the Blind, Hannover, Germany.

Margaret Hills de Zárate is an Art Therapist, Researcher, and Honorary Senior Lecturer in Art Therapy, Queen Margaret University, Edinburgh, UK.

Heather M. Hunter is an Occupational Therapist and Honorary Senior Lecturer in Occupational Therapy, Queen Margaret University, Edinburgh, UK.

Salvo Pitruzzella is a Dramatherapist, Author, and retired Professor of Arts Education, Italy, and Honorary Member of EFD (European Federation of Dramatherapy).

International Research in the Arts Therapies

Series Editors: Diane Waller and Sarah Scoble

A collaboration between ***ECArTE*** *(European Consortium for Arts Therapies Education) and* ***ICRA*** *(International Centre for Research in Arts Therapies)*

This series consists of high-level monographs identifying areas of importance across all arts therapy modalities (art therapy, dance-movement therapy, dramatherapy and music therapy) and highlighting international developments and concerns. It presents recent research from countries across the world and contributes to the evidence-base of the arts therapies. Papers which discuss and analyse current innovations and approaches in the arts therapies and arts therapy education are also included.

This series is accessible to practitioners of the arts therapies and to colleagues in a broad range of related professions, including those in countries where arts therapies are still emerging. The monographs should also provide a valuable source of reference to government departments and health services.

Titles in the Series

Intercultural Arts Therapies Research
Issues and Methodologies
Edited by Ditty Dokter and Margaret Hills de Zárate

Art Therapies and New Challenges in Psychiatry
Edited by Karin Dannecker

Arts Therapies in the Treatment of Depression
Edited by Ania Zubala and Vicky Karkou

Arts Therapies and Gender Issues
International Perspectives on Research
Edited by Susan Hogan

Arts Therapies and the Mental Health of Children and Young People
Contemporary Research, Theory, and Practice, Volume 1
Edited by Uwe Herrmann, Margaret Hills de Zárate, and Salvo Pitruzzella

Arts Therapies Research and Practice with Persons on the Autism Spectrum
Colourful Hatchlings
Edited by Supritha Aithal and Vicky Karkou

Arts Therapies and the Mental Health of Children and Young People
Contemporary Research, Theory, and Practice, Volume 2
Edited by Uwe Herrmann, Margaret Hills de Zárate, Heather M. Hunter, and Salvo Pitruzzella

For more information about the series, including how to contribute, please visit www.routledge.com/ https://www.routledge.com/International-Research-in-the-Arts-Therapies/book-series/IRAT

Arts Therapies and the Mental Health of Children and Young People

Contemporary Research, Theory, and Practice, Volume 2

Edited by Uwe Herrmann, Margaret Hills de Zárate, Heather M. Hunter, and Salvo Pitruzzella

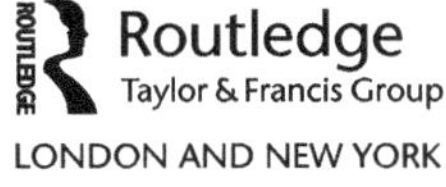
LONDON AND NEW YORK

Designed cover image: *The Storm* (2023) by Solomiya Sles

First published 2024
by Routledge
4 Park Square, Milton Park, Abingdon, Oxon OX14 4RN

and by Routledge
605 Third Avenue, New York, NY 10158

Routledge is an imprint of the Taylor & Francis Group, an informa business

British Library Cataloguing-in-Publication Data
A catalogue record for this book is available from the British Library

Library of Congress Cataloguing-in-Publication Data
Names: Herrmann, Uwe (Art therapist), editor. | Hills De Zárate, Margaret, 1958- editor. | Hunter, Heather M., editor. | Pitruzzella, Salvo, editor.
Title: Arts therapies and the mental health of children and young people : contemporary research, theory and practice. Volume 2 / edited by Uwe Herrmann, Margaret Hills de Zárate, Heather M. Hunter and Salvo Pitruzzella.
Description: Abingdon, Oxon ; New York, NY : Routledge, 2024. |
Series: International research in the arts therapies | Includes bibliographical references and index. |
Identifiers: LCCN 2023041421 (print) | LCCN 2023041422 (ebook) |
ISBN 9781032182940 (hardback) | ISBN 9781032208749 (paperback) |
ISBN 9781003265610 (ebook)
Subjects: LCSH: Art therapy for children. | Art therapy for teenagers. | Art therapy for youth. | Child mental health. | Teenagers--Mental health. | Youth--Mental health.
Classification: LCC RJ505.A7 A793 2024 (print) | LCC RJ505.A7 (ebook) |
DDC 618.92/85882065156--dc23/eng/20231211
LC record available at https://lccn.loc.gov/2023041421
LC ebook record available at https://lccn.loc.gov/2023041422

ISBN: 978-1-032-18294-0 (hbk)
ISBN: 978-1-032-20874-9 (pbk)
ISBN: 978-1-003-26561-0 (ebk)

DOI: 10.4324/9781003265610

Typeset in Sabon
by MPS Limited, Dehradun

The Open Access version of chapter 11 was funded by Dov Blum-Yazdi.

Contents

Note on the cover

Solomiya, a young girl from Ukraine, drew this picture in a nine-month art therapy studio project in Hannover, Germany. The project, conceived by art therapist Uwe Herrmann, was designed for children aged 6–12 who had fled from war-struck Ukraine.

The Storm powerfully and symbolically conveys what the experience of war, displacement, and transition to another country can mean to a child. In this picture, a safe harbour was not yet in sight. In another, but later, version of the same theme, a green, safe, and peaceful shore was well within reach.

Many of the children referred to in this book are facing 'the storm,' be it that they, like Solomiya, have experienced war and persecution or are in transit with no clear destination in sight. Others are marginalised through poverty or discrimination, living with a terminal illness, or enduring invasive medical treatments. Solomiya's image speaks to them all.

Contributors

Mitsi Akoyunoglou is an Assistant Professor of Music Therapy at the Department of Music Studies at Ionian University. She holds a PhD in Music Therapy from Ionian University and completed postdoctoral research on the role of the female lamenter in the individual and collective pain of loss. She has a Bachelor in Music Therapy and a Master in Music Therapy (as a "Onassis Foundation" Scholarship recipient) from Michigan State University, USA. She has a piano diploma from the Athenaeum International Conservatory. She is the Europe regional liaison for the World Federation of Music Therapy (WFMT), the representative of the Hellenic Association of Certified Professional Music Therapists (ESPEM) at the European Confederation of Music Therapy, and a certified supervisor of ESPEM. She is a member of the scientific committee of the journal *Mousikopaidagwgika* [Music Pedagogy] and a member of the editorial board of *Approaches: An Interdisciplinary Journal of Music Therapy*. Her research interests include music therapy, music pedagogy, lamentation and grief, non-formal music teaching practices, music and Universal Design for Learning (UDL), community music and community music therapy with refugee children and adolescents.

Vicky G. Armstrong, PhD, qualified as an art psychotherapist in 2008 and began working with children who had experienced early relational trauma. Armstrong developed a model for parent-infant art therapy groups funded by a series of grants from the Kerr-Fry Trust (2013, 2015) and collaborated with developmental psychologist Dr Josephine Ross to found Art at the Start. This project investigates the impact of early art experiences on the health, wellbeing, and relationships of parents and infants. Armstrong joined the psychology department at the University of Dundee in 2018 as a post-graduate researcher in a funded collaboration with the Dundee Contemporary Arts (DCA) centre to develop this work. Art at the Start is interested in outcomes from participative arts within the DCA gallery and art therapy groups specifically targeting vulnerable parent-infant dyads. Armstrong runs public drop-in sessions in the DCA, offering art and sensory play with parents with babies, toddlers, and preschoolers. She is currently running a large, controlled trial to measure the outcomes of 12-week art therapy groups for parents and infants, which involves participant referrals from health and voluntary services where there are concerns about these early relationships. This trial involves collecting data on attachments and mental wellbeing before and after the art therapy groups and using an observational tool to examine potential changes in behaviour to evaluate the role of art and art psychotherapy in parent-infant relationships.

Diedré M. Blake received a bachelor's degree in studio art from Stanford University (2000) and a master's degree in expressive therapy and clinical mental health counselling, specialising in art therapy, from Lesley University (2006). Her research interests include eating disorders, identity and language acquisition, and acculturation. Currently, she lives in Japan, where she works in education and practises flower arrangement.

Dov Blum-Yazdi, PhD, is a Drama Therapist and Clinical Criminologist. He is a graduate of the psychotherapy mind-body-spirit programme of the University of Haifa, whose doctoral studies were in psychoanalysis and hermeneutics at Bar-Ilan University. In addition, he studies Spiritual Care and Chaplaincy (palliative) at Shutafim Lamasa Association. Dov is a senior supervisor and lecturer in Arts Therapist training programmes at the University of Haifa and Tel Hai Academic College. In addition, he is a Drama Therapist for high school youth groups within the Merhav program in the Ministry of Education, in the position of specialist of group therapy.

Furthermore, Dov owns 'Place to Be,' a drama and art therapy studio; he serves as the international representative of the Israeli division of drama therapists in Yahat and is a peace activist. Dov is the founder and researcher of 'The Leelah Play': 'The Leelah Play paradigm'—Theoretical Concepts of Power, Identity, and Liberty in the Therapeutic Playing Field; and 'Leelah – Play for Itself'—a non-directive model. His current developing and continued research of The Leelah Play is undertaken within his Post-doctoral at the Laboratory of Psychology, University of Crete. For more details, please visit www.leelahplay.com.

Maika Campo, BA in Psychology from the University of the Basque Country (San Sebastian, Spain) in 2001. Master's degree in Dance Movement Therapy (DMT) from the Autonomous University of Barcelona (Barcelona, Spain) in 2010. Maika is a registered member of the Spanish DMT Association and has been a Community Worker in an Educational Centre for Young Offenders since 2006 and involved in DMT workshops for women engaged in migration projects and empowerment activities from 2011 to 2015. In addition, she has been a member of the Master's in Dance Movement Therapy educational team at the Autonomous University of Barcelona since 2014 and published on DMT with Young Offenders.

Chien-Yueh Chiang is a registered art psychotherapist who graduated from Queen Margaret University College in 2014. Since then, she has worked as an art therapist at the Children's Hospital of China Medical University in Taiwan. Her main focus is helping children in the haematology and oncology ward and providing outpatient services in the Division of Child and Adolescent Development and Mental Health. In addition to her work at the hospital, Chien-Yueh Chiang collaborates with the Taichung City Family Violence and Sexual Assault Prevention Centre to provide services at the Child and Adolescent Protection Medical Demonstration Centre. Her dedication to helping children and families affected by violence and trauma is a testament to her passion for improving the lives of others through the therapeutic power of art.

Tina Y. Chu is a registered art psychotherapist with the HCPC (Health & Care Professions Council). She completed a Bachelor of Arts in Fine Art from the University of California Los Angeles in 2002 and a Master's in Art Psychotherapy Practice from the Art Therapy Northern Programme at Leeds Metropolitan University in 2010. Tina's private practice focuses on working with neurotic adult clients and children from high-risk and divorced families in addition to her therapy work. Tina is also the owner of a children's bookshop in Taiwan, which operates on the philosophy of promoting the mental well-being of children with book selection that addresses different psychological needs of children.

Malcy Duff is a cartoonist, art therapist, and performer from Edinburgh, Scotland. His comix include 'The Liminal Sneeze,' 'The Pineapple,' 'The Heroic Mosh of Mary's Son,' and 'A 52 Second Silence for Topsy.' His work has been published in various magazines and anthologies, including MAP, The Wire, Giant Tank Offline, Product, Art Review, and The Comics Journal. He plays and records in the duo Usurper and has been performing his 'live comics' since 2010. Malcy has been developing an approach using comic book storytelling as narrative art therapy. He is currently offering sessions in Comix Art Therapy for children and young people experiencing issues with their mental health in community settings in Edinburgh.

Gloria Garbujo practices Dramatherapy at Shooting Star Children's Hospices, where she leads the service's online Dramatherapy programme with children, young people, and their parents. Gloria is a senior therapist involved in addressing and responding to the changing needs of children and young people in clinical practice. Her academic background is in philosophy, and she collaborates with the University of Padua (Italy), lecturing on the arts therapies in palliative care. As a published author and a bereavement specialist, Gloria is an Associate Supervisor for Talking Heads and Education Support and provides online supervision for school leaders. After ten years of clinical practice in the United Kingdom, Gloria is currently based in Italy, where she leads specialist bereavement courses for mental health professionals.

Claire M. Ghetti, PhD, MT-BC, CCLS, is an Associate Professor of Music Therapy at The Grieg Academy, Department of Music, University of Bergen, Norway, and an Assistant Leader of the Grieg Academy Music Therapy Research Centre (GAMUT), a twin-centre collaboration between the University of Bergen and NORCE Norwegian Research Centre AS. Claire's research centres on how music and the relationships enabled through music serve as resources that can help buffer against traumatisation in intensive medical contexts. She is currently the Principal Investigator of a multinational, randomised controlled trial funded by the Research Council of Norway (LongSTEP, RCN 273534) evaluating the impact of music therapy on longer-term outcomes of parent-infant bonding, infant development, and parental mental health in premature infants and their caregivers. The music therapy approach in LongSTEP is unique in its resource-oriented approach to family-centred care in neonatal contexts, where parents are supported by a trained music therapist to use their innate resources to the mutual benefit of parent and infant alike. Claire has published research and theoretical work in music therapy as procedural support for invasive medical procedures, music therapy for hospitalised children at risk for traumatisation, and music therapy as emotional-approach coping to improve peri-procedural outcomes. As a music therapist and certified child life specialist, Claire has pioneered music therapy programming within paediatric intensive care and neonatal intensive care. She has additional research interests in paediatric palliative care, non-pharmacological treatment of pain and anxiety, and family-centred therapy within medical contexts. Claire holds a PhD in music therapy with a minor in health psychology from the University of Kansas.

Uwe Herrmann (**Editor**) trained in fine art and social pedagogy in Germany and art psychotherapy at the University of Hertfordshire and Goldsmiths College, University of London (PhD). In 1991, he developed the art therapy service at the State Training Institute for the Blind in Hanover, Germany, where he continues his practice with blind and partially sighted children, adolescents, and young adults. Uwe built up Germany's first MA programme in art therapy with Prof. Dr Karin Dannecker at Weissensee Academy of Art Berlin, where he was appointed professor in art therapy in 2014. He has published and lectured widely on art therapy in Germany, many countries of the European Union, the UK, and South Korea. His research interests are the psychodynamics of vision and congenital blindness, symbol formation, and visual/artistic methods of enquiry in art psychotherapy.

Margaret Hills de Zárate (Editor), PhD, is an Honorary Senior Lecturer at Queen Margaret University, Edinburgh, where she taught from 1994–2020 and held the role of programme leader from 2006 to 2016. She initially studied fine art and later trained as an Art Therapist at Goldsmith's College, University of London. Following this, she worked in social work in the public sector. She continued her professional development at the Scottish Institute of Human Relations in psychodynamic counselling and group work while completing her M.Ed at the University of Edinburgh. Her research interests in ethnography, migration, refugee studies, and translation have been supported by her involvement in one of three large grants awarded under the AHRC's Translating Cultures scheme. Margaret has taught extensively in Europe, Latin America, Africa, and India and continues to dedicate her time to research, editing, and voluntary work both in the UK and abroad.

Sarah Hodkinson practises as a Music Therapist at Shooting Star Children's Hospices, where she is the clinical lead and Head of the Family Support Service. Her leadership and development work explores the need and effectiveness of psychosocial support in anticipatory grief and childhood bereavement. Sarah is a Principal Teaching Fellow at the University of Southampton, lecturing in music therapy and leading this curriculum. Sarah engages in research focused on paediatric palliative care and the therapeutic use of music in cochlear implant rehabilitation. Utilising her extensive experience as a practitioner and academic, Sarah works internationally as part of a steering group introducing therapeutic music in Moldova, supporting the de-institutionalisation of existing social-care systems through providing training for those working with children with disabilities.

Heather M. Hunter (Editor), PhD, is an Honorary Senior Lecturer in Occupational Therapy in the Division of Nursing, Occupational Therapy and Arts Therapies at Queen Margaret University, Edinburgh. She trained in Psychoanalytic Group Work, Infant Observation, and Therapeutic Skills with Children and Young People at the Scottish Institute of Human Relations. She worked as an occupational therapist in adult mental health and Child and Adolescent Mental Health Services (CAMHS) for many years. She completed her Master's in Education at the University of Edinburgh and is a Senior Fellow of the Higher Education Academy. Her doctoral studies (PhD) explore how volunteering through personal choice may impact people's lives, using Participatory Action Research (PAR) with people with lived experience of mental illness. Heather holds a public appointment with the Scottish Government as a judicial general member of the Mental Health Tribunal for Scotland, where she is involved in making decisions about the formal detention of individuals, including children and young people, under the Mental Health (Care and Treatment) (Scotland) Act 2003.

Anshuma Kshetrapal is a practising Psychotherapist and a Drama and Movement Therapist. She has an MA in Psychosocial Clinical Studies and another in Drama and Movement Therapy (Sesame). She is a Founding Board Member and Vice President of the Indian Association of Dance Movement Therapy and holds the same position in Drama-Therapy India. In both associations, she is also part of the Ethics Committees. She is a past Honorary Advisory Board Member of the 'Creative Movement Therapy Association of India.' Anshuma is an educator and supervisor for multiple arts therapies courses across India and gives workshops and lectures across India. She's also a curriculum designer, academic consultant, and co-director of the PG Diploma in Dance Movement Therapy. Besides this, she's the founder of The Colour of Grey Cells and co-founder of The Arts Therapists Co-Lab, which provides accessible mental health and works in mental health advocacy through her organisations. Her podcast, 'Mann ki ABC,' produced by Hindustan Times, aims to promote conversations around mental health in Hindi.

Hsiao-Pin Lin completed a master's art therapy degree at Queen Margaret University College in 2004. Pin is a registered art therapist, the former president, and a certified supervisor of the Taiwan Art Therapy Association (TATA). Over the past 19 years, Pin has lectured and led workshops around Taiwan while working with toddlers, children, and adults in Hospitals and NGOs. She is also a promoter of the National Creative Arts Therapy License in Taiwan.

Heidrun Panhofer, PhD, has directed the Master in Dance Movement Therapy at the Department for Clinical Psychology of the Autonomous University of Barcelona, Spain, since 2003. In addition, she teaches and supervises the same programme and also internationally. Heidrun is one of the co-founders, former President, and supervising member of the Spanish Association of Dance Movement Therapy (ADMTE). She has published extensively on Embodied Perceptional Practices, DMT training, Clinical Supervision, different client populations, Interculturality, and Movement Observation and Analysis. Heidrun holds a PhD from the University of Hertfordshire, UK, a master's degree in Dance Movement

Therapy from the Laban Centre for Movement and Dance in London, a diploma in dance from the Scoil Stiofan Naofa in Cork, Ireland, and a degree in Special Education from the Pädagogische Hochschule in Graz, Austria.

Rita Pirovano graduated with honours in developmental Neuro-Psychomotricity. She worked first in a Nursery School and, since 2010, at the Institute of Neuropsychiatry for children and adolescents at the 'Villa Santa Maria' in Tavernerio (CO). For five years, she has been engaged in an experimental project of prevention and well-being by screening children in Jewish kindergartens in Milan, Turin, Florence, Trieste, and Rome. Co-author of the handbook Psychomotor Health, published in 2015. In 2018, she graduated in Dramatherapy at the Centro ArtiTerapie in Lecco with a dissertation focused on dramatherapy with ASD children and adolescents.

Salvo Pitruzzella (Editor) is a pioneer of dramatherapy in Italy. In 1998, he founded Italy's first dramatherapy training course at the Centro ArtiTerapie in Lecco. Until his retirement in 2022, he had been a Tenured Professor of Arts Education at the Fine Arts Academy of Palermo, Italy, where he still teaches Creative Writing. He is one of the founders of the EFD (European Federation of Dramatherapy). He has been a member of the Federation's Executive Board from 2013 to 2023 when he was appointed Member of Honour. Salvo has written and edited many books on dramatherapy, creativity, arts education, and applied theatre, including *Drama, Creativity and Intersubjectivity: Foundations of Change in Dramatherapy*, London & New York, Routledge, 2016. He has also published three novels and the first Italian translation of William Blake's poem *Vala, or The Four Zoas.* (https://sites.google.com/view/spitruzzelladramatherapy/home-page)

Preetha Ramasubramanian is a Dance Movement Psychotherapist (DMP) who graduated from Goldsmiths College, University of London, and is practising in India. She has an M.Sc. in Psychology from the University of Madras and a PG Dip in Special Education. Preetha is a PhD candidate enroled at the University of Hertfordshire, UK. Preetha is the Co-Founder and President of the Indian Association of Dance Movement Therapy (IADMT) and a past Honorary Advisory Board Member for the Creative Movement Therapy Association of India. She co-founded 'The Arts Therapists Co-Lab' (TATC), which promotes well-being, by conducting training programmes, workshops, and masterclasses for students, therapists, and clients across India. Preetha is a co-director of the PG Diploma in DMT. She also teaches and supervises other PG Diploma Courses, and is invited as a guest lecturer at various universities across

India, and acts as a consultant conducting group/individual sessions and workshops in various institutions.

Giorgos Tsiris, PhD, is Director of Education, Research and Creative Arts at St Columba's Hospice Care and Senior Lecturer in Music Therapy at Queen Margaret Universityin Edinburgh, Scotland. Since 2009, Giorgos has been working as a music therapist in palliative care. He has led award-winning health promotion and death education initiatives disrupting societal attitudes towards death, dying and loss. His doctoral research was an ethnographic study of spirituality in everyday music therapy contexts, and his research portfolio covers a range of areas including service evaluation and professionalisation issues in the arts therapies. Giorgos is co-editor-in-chief of *Approaches: An Interdisciplinary Journal of Music Therapy* – a bilingual (English-Greek) open access publication – and co-author of two books on service evaluation and research ethics respectively. He has served as the representative of the Hellenic Association of Certified Professional Music Therapists (ESPEM) at the European Music Therapy Confederation, and co-chaired the 2022 European Music Therapy Conference in the UK.

Introduction

Salvo Pitruzzella, Heather M. Hunter, Margaret Hills de Zárate, and Uwe Herrmann

This second volume of collected papers expands on the first, with the aim of enlarging the horizon of contemporary and innovative research, practice, and theory in the arts therapies, addressing the mental health of children and young people from an international perspective. Offering a widened range of perspectives, this book adds to the kaleidoscope of possibilities offered by the creative approach of the arts therapies and of the manifold ways in which the different languages of the arts may meet the needs of children and adolescents.

This volume presents diverse perspectives, addressing different client groups and settings. It reports experiences in a variety of contexts where the modalities of dance, music, drama, and art therapies are applied. Chapters range from the introduction of music therapy with refugee children in Greece to the Dance Movement Therapy with a victim of sexual abuse in a Spanish detention centre. It reports experiences with pre-adolescents with ASD spectrum, LGBTQIA+ young people in residential settings, children in hospices, and paediatric medical hospitals. Contributions address how early Arts Therapies interventions may prevent insecure and ambivalent attachment, propose new creative methods of working, and offer interesting insights into childhood and adolescence in different cultures through the lens of their specific cultural and creative approaches. From the variety of approaches, some significant themes emerge, which invite further exploration. While the chapters report different forms of evidence drawn upon experience gathered from practice and research, in all of them, the artistic perspective is paramount. This means that some shared understandings intrinsic to all artistic phenomena inform our ways of thinking and acting therapeutically, the first of which is creativity. As the dramatherapist Robert Landy suggested, if we aim at reawakening the creative abilities of our clients, we must 'embody the creative principle and mirror it, to return it back on the client' (cited in Jennings ed. 1992, p. 110). Creativity includes three main attitudes, which are rooted in the ways children encounter the world and can be nurtured throughout life: *Curiosity, Versatility*, and *Presence*. 'Curiosity is a way of turning towards the world, of meeting experience. Versatility is a way of considering the world, of contacting experience. Presence is a way of being

DOI: 10.4324/9781003265610-1

in the world, of living experience' (Pitruzzella, 2016, p. 80). The chapters explore new territories, which implies facing the unexpected. This entails encouraging young clients' ability to wonder, to improvise, to grasp new chances in what may be upsetting, and follow spontaneity and the fire of the moment.

Most importantly, this means being able 'to accept momentary ambivalences and ambiguities, enduring moments of chaos and confusion' (ibid.). To live through such moments, young clients need the presence of someone who knows how to be with them while not being them and who finds the right distance to create a caring relationship. It involves attention to the here and now and aesthetic sensibility to foster awareness of what Daniel Stern (2004) called 'Now Moments' and simultaneously develop or maintain a reflective stance.

The book opens with a chapter by Vicky Armstrong on infancy and early childhood, where the foundations are laid for every aspect of human development, including physical, intellectual, emotional, and mental health (Marmot, 2010). It is recognised that around 250 million children worldwide may not reach their developmental potential due to health, nutritional, and psychosocial risks, and interventions targeting the first three years of life when the brain is sensitive to the environment and experiences are particularly effective in improving cognitive, language, and motor skills, as well as socio-emotional development and attachment (Jeong et al., 2021). Significantly, interventions targeting responsive caregiving have been found to have greater effects on child developmental outcomes than those interventions with no responsive caregiving content (ibid.). This chapter draws on Armstrong's ground-breaking Art at the Start project in Dundee, Scotland, promoting art-making between caregivers and their infants to improve early childhood development in keeping with the World Health Organisation's (2020) objective to identify early child development evidence-based specific interventions and feasible approaches that are effective in improving developmental outcomes in children (p. viii). It investigates the impact of early art experiences on the health, well-being, and relationships within the vulnerable dyad of caregiver and infant from an art therapy perspective. This contribution reinforces the value of shared art-making as an early intervention to follow and respond to their infant's lead within a safe and supportive environment. Case vignettes illustrate how art therapy can facilitate positive communication and attachment through joint attention, attunement, physical contact, and attention to the art-making process and the qualities of the materials employed.

The following chapter by Mitsi Akoyunoglou and Giorgos Tsiris describes a five-year practice-led exploration of group music therapy with refugee children on the Greek island of Chios, which draws upon Akoyunoglou's ethnographic field notes recorded in situ. Ethnographers are interested in what people have in their minds and what they do as a holistic and dialectical way of understanding human beings. It focuses on complexity and people and has been described as the most humanistic of the social sciences and the most scientific of the humanities (Demossier, in Wall et al., 2018). An inductive approach, such as ethnography, allows the researcher flexibility and, therefore, to respond to situations in the context in which the research is being undertaken is demonstrated in this chapter. This account of music therapy practice makes an important contribution, as the literature on therapeutic work within transit camps, used as temporary shelters for new arrivals to provide short-term temporary accommodation for displaced populations, is to date limited. This chapter outlines the development of a community-oriented approach to music therapy and the everyday refugee experience within formal and informal transit camps, explored and underpinned by the principles of Psychological First Aid (PFA), the wider community, and the role of music therapy in supporting refugee children's experience of crisis and adversity.

A further example of how the Arts Therapies support resilience in children facing adversities can be found in Chapter 3, where music therapist Sarah Hodkinson and dramatherapist Gloria Garbujo present their work in a children's hospice. In the previous chapter, music therapy has been shown to be effective in helping children to cope with the stress caused by the traumatic changes they have endured. It contributes to creating, in people who are 'in limbo,' a sense of community, which can foster hope for the future. Hodkinson and Garbujo describe a context that is another sort of limbo; the life-limiting conditions of the hospice patient have removed them from the outside world and made them dependent on the care of other people. The medical therapies they undergo cannot promise to heal, only relieve them from the worst symptoms and slow down the inevitable progression of their terminal condition. Under these conditions, ideas of 'future' or 'hope' may be compromised, and any intervention might only offer moments of distraction from their persistent symptoms and terminal condition. The authors demonstrate that the arts can do more than this: they can provide children with moments to fully enjoy their lives. Two case vignettes demonstrate how songwriting and storytelling enabled therapist and client to establish a safe and warm relationship where creativity can flow. Aldo Carotenuto maintained that 'the meaning of creativity does not have to be necessarily associated to the great artistic expressions, but to the fact that a single being can succeed in experimenting with new things, in building within one's own experience a life dimension in which the same drive that led or pushed Leonardo, Michelangelo, Beethoven or Proust, to create, can be active' (Carotenuto, 1991, p. 552).

In Chapter 4, Hsiao-Pin Lin, Teena Y. Chu, and Chien-Yueh Chiang introduce a different cultural point of view on childhood, looking at the role of grandparents as primary caregivers for their grandchildren as an increasingly common global phenomenon (Bai et al., 2023). The authors explore the influence of multigenerational relationships on Taiwanese children through art therapy and object relations theory. They explain how Taiwan's diverse communities have adopted the cultural principle and ethical concept of filial piety, where grandparents are accorded absolute authority. The chapter adopts an attachment perspective to understand the dynamics of art therapy with children in intergenerational households. Three case vignettes explore how the role of grandparents may impact the children and the parent-child relationship. The authors conclude that while the quality of object relations and filial piety determined how each child responded to fraught family relationships, separation, absence, and loss, the art-making process and the 'as if' function of symbolisation constituted powerful agents in the therapeutic process.

In Chapter 5, Claire M. Ghetti considers the unique and pioneering contributions from a Norwegian perspective on music therapy practice in intensive paediatric medical contexts. Adopting a socioecological lens and drawing on key theoretical constructs illustrated through case material, Ghetti invites us to better appreciate the impact of hospitalisation and treatment for severe and life-threatening illness on the child and young person-in-context, where the illness and the nested social structures that the child is embedded in cannot be separated from each other. In doing so, Ghetti usefully problematises health to reveal an existential understanding of where health and illness co-exist. Music therapy is presented as a process of 'musicking,' an invaluable resource-oriented and salutogenic intervention that supports this existential position and offers a bridge between the micro, meso, and exo-systems of the child's social ecology. Constituting a family-centred way of connecting with innate resources, Ghetti demonstrates how music therapy as a trauma-informed practice supports trauma prevention and protects against the impact of the illness, potential (re-)traumatisation, and further trauma induced by medical treatment procedures in intensive paediatric medical contexts.

Heidrun Panhofer and Maika Campo report and reflect on Dance Movement Therapy (DTM) with child sexual abuse, trauma, and psychosis in Chapter 6. They present a case study on a migrant adolescent offender, abused as a child and who was later prosecuted for perpetrating abuse on a minor and developed a psychotic illness in a centre for offenders.

Dance Movement Therapy was introduced as an intervention to create a safe environment, using embodied perceptual practices, creativity, and bodily movement to contain the boy's fragmented self. For this client, DMT was instrumental in a process enabling him to begin to find his own limits and to separate from his magical inner world that was confusing, fascinating, and frightening. Connecting early sexual trauma and the violation of interpersonal boundaries with dissociative psychotic symptoms, the chapter describes DMT as offering a potential means to find a safe space in which dance, movement, and a secure relationship with the DMT therapist can contribute to a patient's further healing.

In Chapter 7, Preetha Ramasubramanian and Anshuma Kshetrapal provide an insight into developing psychoeducation through dance therapy and dramatherapy for adolescents in urban school settings in India. They describe their project's specific, culturally relevant challenges, demands, and benefits, as well as the intricacies of service development and implementation in the context of Indian health care and education. Their account can be understood as a model case of pioneering arts therapies practice in a social, political, and historical context where practitioners must develop their service in response to clients' needs. Bridging the gap between health care and education, they describe how they had to tailor their work to the parameters of existing service provision, available resources, and the varied cultures and political structures in India.

In Chapter 8, Malcy Duff discusses the therapeutic value of the comic panel in art therapy with children and young people with mental health difficulties in integrated school settings and special schools. The text is illustrated with a series of comic panels that comment on and further illuminate its content, presenting Duff's ideas of the comic panel in practice. In this innovative approach, the comic panel functions as visual communication in which captions may or may not be added as an additional verbal narrative. Drawing on the role of the frame and containment, he explores the connection between the use of the comic panel in a therapeutic space and psychoanalytic theories, for example, Winnicott (2005) and Milner (2013) that have largely influenced art therapy practice and thinking, and Schaverien's (1999) writing in art therapy. Duff concludes with suggestions for further approaches to the use of the comic panel in art therapy practice and their practical applications.

In Chapter 9, Italian dramatherapist Rita Pirovano illustrates her pioneering experience of dramatherapy applied to groups of pre-adolescents with Autistic Spectrum Disorder. The estimated rates of 4–10 children with autism per 10,000 have multiplied tenfold in a few years since 2015. It is unclear whether this increase is due to a broader definition of the disorder at the expense of other pathologies or broader diagnostic criteria, greater awareness of the condition, or an increasingly early diagnosis.

In recent years there has been a growing interest in artistic approaches since the metaphoric-projective dimension provided by the art form seems to be a safe-enough container for children to express themselves. It has been suggested that 'dramatherapy can reach out to people on the autistic spectrum by recognising difference and individuality, and through a broad range of techniques, can support people to express their feelings and imagination, and develop their communication and social skills' (Haythorne & Seymour, 2017, p. 9). Pirovano's chapter inquires into the range of therapeutic factors implicit in the dramatic process, which can address the main impairments present in ASD conditions, namely the lack of interaction, communication, and imagination, which express themselves as difficulties in storytelling, recognition, expression, and management of emotions, poor tolerance for frustration, lack of self-awareness, and rigidity of thought. She compares the growth of children's dramatic skills in the process to the reduction of these impairments, using tools both from dramatherapy and neuropsychiatry, with promising results.

Diedré M. Blake, in Chapter 10, writes retrospectively about having worked in art therapy with LGBTQIA+ youth in residential settings in the North-Eastern United States. She provides insights into the psychological and social challenges this group experiences, particularly individuals coming from diverse social, racial, and cultural backgrounds. The chapter highlights the huge changes the landscape of practice and thinking in this area has undergone. Blake reflects on the practice that she undertook while still in training and draws attention to the fact that this area is still, and increasingly, developing. She discerns five themes of importance in this work that may inform further practice, ranging from social displacement to challenges to finding community, changing self-identification, embracing new modes of self-expression, and the importance of bridging the multicultural gap.

In the final Chapter 11, Dov Blum-Yazdi introduces an innovative model of dramatherapy, which he calls 'The Leelah Play,' inspired by ideas from the Greek Polis and the role-playing game Dungeons & Dragons. Outlining the model's theoretical framework, Blum-Yazdi provides insight into a practice process in which it is applied with a group of young people. Leelah is a Sanskrit term that signifies the eternal play of the Gods, through which the universes are created and destroyed. The author suggests that, in practice, dramatherapy often aims at controlling the play. Rather than letting it flow freely, the dramatherapist wants to direct it towards goals assumed to be for the client's own good, which, according to Blum-Yazdi, disturbs the natural flow of play, jeopardising its inherent healing potential. Therefore, in the presented model, the therapist's role is that of a master of ceremonies: to provide safe boundaries within which play can arise and a few hints about the setting, namely the kind of imaginative world that serves as a narrative background for the roles that people will create. Afterwards, the therapist will withdraw, acting just like an observer and appearing only occasionally in the role of a messenger to summon a village meeting to recapitulate the development of the stories so far. For the rest, people can engage with their roles, relationships, or conflicts without the therapist intervening.

This position prompts another important issue, namely the power relationships in therapy, which Michel Foucault in 1978 warned against, lest therapy would become a process of normalisation, in which the therapist exerts an authority based on knowledge about what is normal that the client cannot question (2007). Leelah's approach cautions against this issue and invites reflection on all the implications of our role as therapists.

The picture that emerges from the positions outlined in these papers is that arts therapists, when working with isolated, pressured, and suffering children and young people, often struggle with unfavourable conditions and professional isolation. They must be resourceful, imaginative, flexible, playful, and inventive when relating to individual clients, groups, or the systems their practice is embedded in. They must be not only firmly rooted in psychotherapy theory and practice but be especially grounded in their respective art form. This book proposes, in multiple ways, that the arts in therapy carry unique possibilities to open up a space for the child to express and resolve conflict, to develop, or find meaning in the moment of art-making and relating to another person, be it the therapist or peers, even within the most limiting parameters. Maybe it is here that we can see most clearly why human beings make art: it is in the act of making and looking at art that we find and confirm our sense of individuality and community, and communicate to others who we are, or as a legacy to who we were.

References

Bai, X., Chen, M., He, R., and Xu, T. (2023). Toward an integrative framework of intergenerational co-parenting within family systems: A scoping review. *Journal of Family Theory & Review*, 15(1), pp. 78–117. 10.1111/jftr.12478

Carotenuto, A. (1991). *Trattato di psicologia della personalità*. Milano: Raffaello Cortina.

Foucault, M. (2007). Security, territory, population, in security, territory, population: Lectures at the College De France, 1977–78. In Arnold I. Davidson and Graham Burchell (Eds), (Translation) *Michel Foucault: Lectures at the Collège de France*. London: Palgrave Macmillan.

Haythorne, D., and Seymour, A. (Eds) (2017). Dramatherapy and autism. In *Dramatherapy and autism*. London: Routledge. 10.4324/9781315733838

Jeong, J., Franchett, E. E., Ramos de Oliveira, C. V. et al. (2021). Parenting interventions to promote early child development in the first three years of life: A global systematic review and meta-analysis. *PLoS Medicine*, 18(5), p. e1003602. 10.1371/journal.pmed.1003602

Landy, R. (1992). One-on-one: The role of the dramatherapist working with individuals. In S. Jennings (Ed), *Dramatherapy. Theory and practice 2*. London: Jessica Kingsley Publishers.

Marmot, M. (2010). Fair society, healthy lives. The Marmot review. *Strategic Review of Health Inequalities in England post-2010*. London.

Milner, M. (2013). Winnicott: Overlapping circles and the two-way journey, a paper presented a memorial meeting for D.W. Winnicott, given to the British Psychoanalytical Society in 1972. In Jan Abram (Ed), *Donald Winnicott Today, the new library of psychoanalysis*. London and New York: Routledge.

Pitruzzella, S. (2016). *Drama, creativity and intersubjectivity: The roots of change in dramatherapy*. New York, NY: Routledge.

Schaverien, J. (1999). *The revealing image: Analytical art psychotherapy in theory and Practice*. London and Philadelphia: Jessica Kingsley Publishers.

Schaverien, J. (1989). The picture within the frame. In A. Gilroy and T. Dalley (Eds), *Pictures at an exhibition*. London: Routledge.

Stern, D. (2004). *The present moment in psychotherapy and everyday life, (Norton Series on Interpersonal Neurobiology)*. New York: W. W. Norton & Company.

Wall, G., Demossier, M., and Hills de Zárate, M. (2018). Looking not for truth but meaning: An introduction to ethnography with Professor Marion Demossier and Dr Margaret Hills de Zárate. *Exchanges: The Interdisciplinary Research Journal*, 5(2), pp. 16–25. Retrieved from: http://exchanges.warwick.ac.uk/index.php/exchanges/article/view/254.

Winnicott, D. W. (1971) 2005. *Playing and reality*, 2nd New York: Routledge.

World Health Organization (2020). Improving early childhood development: WHO guideline. ISBN 978-92-4-000209-8 (electronic version).

Chapter 1

Very early art therapy intervention

Why work with infants and their caregivers?

Vicky G. Armstrong

Introduction

This chapter will examine why and how we might intervene at a very early stage to improve wellbeing and attachment relationships by working creatively with infants and their caregivers together through art therapy. When thinking of infants, I am including babies and toddlers from birth to three years. Through those three years, they are organising their mental picture of the world and *adapting* to it (Winberg, 2005). This makes it even more pressing that we intervene early if their environment, primarily formed by their central relationships, is not meeting their needs. If we can intervene early to improve babies' experiences with their primary attachment figures, then there is potential to have ongoing benefits, given that positive early relational experiences are foundational for the development of emotional wellbeing, capacity to regulate, sense of self and brain development (Svanberg, 1998; Schore, 2001; Sroufe, 2005; Barlow et al., 2016).

The World Health Organization (2020) gives guidance that all infants should receive responsive care during their first three years of life and that parents should be supported to provide this. At present, in the United Kingdom, the picture of support for perinatal and infant mental health from specialist services is extremely variable and particularly limited in Scotland and Northern Ireland (Maternal Mental Health Alliance, 2020). Art therapy could play an important role in increasing such provision. This chapter draws on my work developing the Art at the Start project, which promotes art making between caregivers and their infants in several settings, including art therapy groups (Armstrong, 2021). These have shown that art making can draw dyads into positive interactions and help increase parental responsiveness (Armstrong et al., 2019). Other published case studies have shown similar promising results (Arroyo and Fowler, 2013; Lavey-Khan and Reddick, 2020).

This chapter considers what responsive care looks like and when there is a need for very early intervention in a caregiver-infant relationship. I use the term caregiver, thinking about whomever the primary attachment figure is for the infant. I will explore why an art therapy approach may be beneficial

DOI: 10.4324/9781003265610-2

to relationships, in particular the ways in which the process of making art together may encourage interactive behaviours with the regulative, mind-minded, and nurturing processes known to be key in building positive attachments (De Wolff and van Ijzendoorn, 1997). This theoretical discussion will be grounded in case vignettes from art therapy groups that took place within the Art at the Start project to examine and better understand the ways in which the art making process can facilitate positive early interactions. These vignettes are presented with a description of behaviours observed during the session and then the 'facilitators notes' based on the discussions of the art therapist and co-facilitator as they discuss cases in their shared reflective time. The vignettes are designed to be separate from the main text as an example of how a number of issues from the theoretical discussion may connect to our understanding of parents and infant dyads that we see and how we respond. This chapter will be relevant to the practice of those working with very young children across a range of settings, from statutory health services to community or gallery settings. My focus is on visual art here, but there will be commonality with other creative therapeutic modalities, such as music, play, or relationally focused psychotherapies.

Clinical material has been anonymised, and the work was undertaken with ethics consent from the University of Dundee Ethics Committee.

Responsive early relationships

At its simplest, a secure attachment is one where a baby has learned that when they cry, their caregiver will respond, most of the time, with warmth and reassurance (Benoit, 2004). They feel safe to express a negative emotion and can seek physical proximity to a caregiver. Their expectation is that they will be helped when distressed and that this will make them feel better. In time this expectation of safety will free them up to start exploring their world (Bowlby, 1997).

But early interactions are about more than safety. Babies are born intrinsically able to communicate, actively seeking to connect with others. Trevarthen (2001) calls this primary intersubjectivity. Newborn babies can mimic facial expressions, drawing their caregivers in. The sensitive caregiver responds, beginning a 'conversation.' These conversations become increasingly reciprocal, with a mutually rewarding 'serve and return' rhythm of turn taking, in which the baby uses all their channels of communication, e.g., facial expressions, vocalisations, musicality, bodily gestures, and rhythms. In this way, caregivers do not just soothe their babies; they are also stimulating their babies, 'up-regulating' within pleasurable limits, thus expanding their babies' emotional range with playfulness and positive affect (Stern, 2000; Trevarthen, 2001).

Timing is important in these interactions, with the caregiver's sensitivity allowing for the development of synchrony (Feldman, 2007). Feldman describes how a caregiver is able to pick up on the subtle shifts in their newborn's state of alertness and adapt their own responses accordingly, targeting stimulating interactions when babies shift into a more attentive state. Babies who are securely attached experience more synchronous interactions, which are well timed and mutually rewarding, compared to babies showing insecure attachments where the caregivers may be either under-involved or intrusive (Isabella and Belsky, 1991). But the interactions do not always have to be perfectly timed. Tronick (2007) highlights the patterns of mismatches followed by interactive repairs, which are a feature of normal communications.

Within these synchronous interactions, where caregivers respond contingently to their baby's behaviour, the baby sees that their own actions have made something happen. They learn that they can create a predictable response in their caregiver, the experience of which will develop their sense of self-efficacy (Bigelow et al., 2010). Self-efficacy is foundational for a baby's developing sense of self (Svanberg, 1998). The baby also learns from the caregiver's contingent responses that it is possible to share their own affect state, their inner world, with another person. This relates to the concept of attunement (Stern, 2000), where a caregiver affirms a baby's expression of affect through contingent marked mirroring. This means caregivers return an expression in a different channel, whereby the baby feels they have been understood. These experiences of being related *to*, shape how babies see themselves and relate to others. Children who experience consistent attunement later present with more social skills like empathy (Mikulincer et al., 2005) and have fewer conflicts (Sroufe, 2005).

Within these sensitive communications, caregivers are able to notice and respond when their baby communicates a need. When a baby is upset, and their caregiver responds to calm them, the caregiver has a biological impact, reducing the high cortisol levels released during periods of distress. Left unchecked, high cortisol can have a long-term impact on the baby's sensitivity to stress hormones and the development of their brain, particularly in the frontal cortex (Shonkoff et al., 2012). On a psychosocial level, from that experience of a responsive caregiver offering comfort to distress, babies will, in turn, learn how to manage their own feelings. These relational experiences build babies' capacity for emotional regulation (Sroufe, 2005) and are predictive of later executive function (Bernier et al., 2012).

Much of what happens in these interactions is unconscious on the part of the sensitive caregiver, but they may also more actively wonder about their baby's feelings and experiences. Mind-mindedness is when a sensitive caregiver is able to think about their baby's intentions and see their baby's behaviour as meaningful in the context of an underlying mental state (Meins et al., 2002). It can also be framed as a 'reflective function' or 'mentalisation' (Camoirano, 2017). This capacity in the caregiver allows them to see their baby as an active participant in interactions. When the caregiver responds as if their baby's behaviour has meaning, the baby will also learn to see their own behaviour in this way (Meins et al., 2002).

The last important point to make about these positive early interactions is that they can be protective against later adversity, making them important for all those working therapeutically, whatever their clients' life stages. Secure attachment appears to protect against other risk factors of early childhood, such as economic deprivation, reduced support networks, discrimination, single parent households, and health inequalities (Moullin et al., 2014). Thus, secure attachments increase children's resilience and may also improve outcomes for future generations, given the cyclical nature of attachment difficulties (Steele et al., 1996).

When early relationships are problematic

On the other hand, where these early relationships do not progress well, babies are missing out on these positive experiences of care and connection. Their distress may go unregulated, cues may be missed, babies are not engaged in playful synchronous 'conversations,' and they do not receive the validation of their own experiences and affect through contingent responses. We see wide-ranging impacts on the wellbeing and mental health of children (Belsky, 2001). This includes difficulties processing emotions and in social relationships (Van Der Voort et al., 2014); externalising problems such as aggression or hyperactivity (Fearon et al., 2010); delays in cognitive developments such as language (Murray and Yingling, 2000); and reduced capacity for empathy, compassion, and social conscience (Music, 2011).

It is thought that around 40% of babies do not experience the responsive relationships which build secure attachments (Moullin et al., 2014). A caregiver who is consistently unresponsive to the baby's needs may result in the baby minimising their expressions of need. A caregiver who is sometimes responsive but at other times rejecting may cause a baby to become constantly focused on how to maintain their caregiver's availability. Or, at worst, the caregiver themselves may be the source of the infant's distress if they are frightening or using the baby to meet their own needs (Barlow et al., 2016). We see how these adaptive strategies, based on the baby's expectations of their caregiver, become the well-known attachment patterns of avoidance, ambivalence, and disorganisation (Ainsworth, 1989).

The caregiver's mental health has a demonstrable impact on the attachment process (Cummings and Cicchetti, 1990) and is shown to increase the risk of later social and emotional difficulties (Kingston and Tough, 2014) and impact cognitive development (Grace et al., 2003). Research into caregivers' mental health has primarily focused on mothers, and it has been found that around 20% of women will develop a mental health condition while pregnant or in the first year of their baby's life (Bauer et al., 2014).

Post-natal depression is perhaps the most recognised mental health difficulty affecting new mothers, with universal screening in place in the UK and a large body of research into the potential impact on relationships (Murray et al., 1996). However, barriers remain to accessing support (Goodman, 2009), such as stigma and accessibility. There is increasing recognition of the prevalence of post-partum anxiety and the potentially negative consequences on bonding, interactions, and ongoing development (Field, 2018). There is also developing research into the risks of post-traumatic stress in early motherhood (Harrison et al., 2021). Granat et al. (2017) give a clear example of how maternal mental health impacts the quality of caregiver-baby interactions with the example of synchrony. They found that depressed mothers often presented with a flat affect, offering less opportunity for the relational sequences of serve-and-return to develop with their babies. At the same time, they found that anxious mothers may offer positive social cues, such as smiling, but 'miss-time' them so that they do not respond to the infant's attentive moments. In missing these chances, their babies will miss rewarding and affirming interpersonal communications.

Evidence of similar mental health difficulties for new fathers, and the impact of this on their babies, is also growing (Habib, 2012), with one in ten new fathers thought to experience depression (Williams, 2020). Johansson et al. (2020) found that depression for mothers and fathers affected their spousal relationships and increased loneliness, potentially also reducing the caregivers' support systems within the family.

In addition to mental health difficulties triggered by birth or parenthood, there may also be pre-existing mental health conditions for caregivers which impact early relationships. Some of these may increase in severity around the perinatal period or may be risk factors for developing perinatal mental health difficulties (O'Hara and Wisner, 2014). One of the most prevalent risk factors for early relationship difficulties is a parent's own experience of attachment (Steele et al., 1996). There may also be social circumstances such as deprivation, isolation, or domestic violence that preoccupy the caregiver, leaving them less emotionally available to pick up the subtle interactional cues from their infant. It is important to consider the intersectionality between mental health, life experiences, and social inequalities, with caregivers who face socio-economic inequalities at higher risk of developing perinatal mental illness (Ban et al., 2012). The strong link between social inequalities and parent-infant health is demonstrated by the persistent and intergenerational nature of parental and child mental health disparities (Klawetter and Frankel, 2018).

Early intervention in relationships

Acquarone (2004) points out that while the caregiver's mental health may be improved with longer-term psychotherapy intervention, the parent-infant relationship cannot wait for this. It is both important and efficacious to intervene early in the relationship. Dyadic intervention, where the relationship is the focus of the therapy, can be seen as a very direct way to improve interactions (Baradon, 2005). This focus on parent-infant relationships is also supported by evidence suggesting that improvement in the quality of attachment relationships may have a mitigating effect on the impact of a caregiver's poor post-natal mental health (Bergman et al., 2010). A review of interventions for infants whose caregivers were experiencing mental health difficulties (Newton et al., 2022) found a number of common approaches behind successful interventions, which included facilitating positive interactions, helping caregivers to see things from the baby's perspective, and using video to give feedback.

Interventions may focus on building the caregiver's reflective function (Suchman et al., 2011; Camoirano, 2017) with the intention that more insight into their infant's feelings and behaviours will allow for more sensitive responses. Video feedback may be used to help caregivers view interactions from their infant's perspective, often with a focus on building on positive moments (Jones, 2006). Programmes such as Watch, Wait, Wonder (Cohen et al., 1999) take an infant-led approach where caregivers are encouraged to follow their infant's spontaneous communications, emphasising the physical availability of the caregiver. This approach, which focuses on following infant-initiated interactions rather than on the parent's perceptions, may be more effective in directly influencing the quality of interactions. In a controlled trial of parent-infant psychotherapy, Fonagy et al. (2016) found that the main effects were on the mother's own mental health and her perceptions of her infant rather than seeing a change in the parent-infant interactions. A review of over 70 different intervention studies found that the clearest benefits to parent-child interactions were in those interventions which took an active, behavioural focused approach (Bakermans-Kranenburg et al., 2003). This steer towards interventions which actively focus on encouraging the caregiver to follow and respond to their infant's lead is one which strongly supports the approach taken within parent-infant art therapy.

Vignette—Mum and Leanne

A young mother and her daughter Leanne, 20 months, are painting together on the floor. In previous sessions, the art therapists held concerns that, while enthusiastic about the art making process, mum can often be more focused on her own making than on the interaction with her daughter. Perhaps she has missed out on some of these experiences in her own early years. Or perhaps she is anxious to be seen to be good at it by the art therapist or the rest of the group—she does often seem demonstrative in her behaviour. Sometimes it feels as if she is relating to Leanne more as an object than as an individual with her own inner world and intentions—for example, picking her up without asking and putting her into a box to take a photo or painting onto Leanne's face. In this session, though, the art therapist is pleased to see them engaged in some shared attention as they both paint together on the same piece of paper. Interestingly this session is quieter, with several parents late to join. They are sitting together on the floor with Leanne in front, between her mum's legs. They start trying out some stamps together, pressing them into paint and then onto the page. Mum then begins to turn to the side and loses some connection as she starts to stamp on her own page. Leanne dips a brush in the paint and starts to paint colour onto the sole of her own foot. The art therapist observed to Mum how Leanne has remembered doing this and learned that it's something we do here. Mum and another parent both comment on how clever Leanne is, and Mum enjoys this praise for her daughter. Mum still does not quite join with her daughter in the activity. The art therapist 'speaks through the baby,' who is trying to get the bottom of her own foot in the paint, observing that it looks as if she needs Mum's help to get those tricky bits. Mum asks if she wants help and takes the brush to paint her foot. Leanne holds her hand to stand up and balances on one foot to make the print.

Facilitators' notes

Mum had found it hard to be present for Leanne in the space. She has a history of anxiety, exacerbated following the birth of Leanne. She feels very performative to us rather than focused on Leanne, and we wonder if she is worried about how she is perceived. Is she scanning the room to assess how safe she is and needs to be vigilant in front of the other mums in the group and us? We wonder if being a young single parent makes her feel more judged by society and exaggerates this. This week felt like a bit of a breakthrough, and maybe the lower numbers at the start meant she felt less pressure to perform. The activity this week also seemed to have engaged them both, and there was a nice feeling of closeness that had not been there in previous weeks. In commenting on the foot painting, we were seeking to highlight a positive, that the baby has remembered a previous positive experience here, as well as encouraging mum to reflect. In this instance, that did not seem to regain Mum's focus, and so we were more direct, voicing Leanne. Mum was able to respond to this and join in. This shift into more shared play, and Mum being more able to reflect on what Leanne needed, was sustained throughout the following weeks. It was also nice to see Mum supporting others in the group in later weeks, encouraging them to try things.

Art in early relationship interventions

Given that the baby is preverbal, the dynamics of early relationships are played out through the physical and visual cues of the interaction, so arts therapies, where the visual and physical activity of art making is an integral component, are innately suited. The UK All-Party Report on Arts in Health and Wellbeing (2017) highlighted the use of arts to improve health and wellbeing of parent-infant dyads in a participative arts context. There are a number of examples from this field of art interventions for mothers (Hogan, 2015) and for parents and infants together (Black et al., 2015; Hibbins and Turner, 2020). Art therapy is an intervention which uses all the benefits of the art making process, but it also offers the safety created by a facilitator who, as a qualified art therapist, has an in-depth understanding of mental health and attachments and who is trained to create a safe space and offer support and containment. In the following discussion, I will be looking at beneficial qualities inherent within the art making process, available in art therapy, as well as qualities about making art in the specific context of art therapy with the presence of a psychotherapist.

While art therapists may draw on traditional techniques from parent-infant psychotherapy for encouraging caregivers to recognise and respond to babies' communications, such as 'voicing the baby,' the art process provides additional opportunities to engage caregivers and create change by directly altering behaviour. A review of art therapy with parents and infants found that the capacity to bring dyads together into positive interactions was central (Armstrong and Ross, 2020). There are now a number of published case studies of art therapy focusing on the parent-infant relationship (Proulx, 2002; Hall, 2008; Parashak, 2008; Armstrong and Howatson, 2015; Hosea, 2017; Meyerowitz-Katz, 2017; Bruce, 2020). Three studies used standardised outcome measures, which found improvements in parental wellbeing and in the parents' perception of the relationship (Arroyo and Fowler, 2013; Armstrong et al., 2019; Lavey-Khan and Reddick, 2020). Another set of case studies describes art therapy where the intervention is focused on the parents' mental health or their mental representations of their infant, with varying inclusion of the infant in the process (Perry et al., 2008; Rayment, 2017; Xeros-Constantinides et al., 2017; Bruce and Hackett, 2020). There is a clear overlap in the aims and application of these approaches, but the discussion below focuses on dyadic work with art therapy as a relationship intervention; in particular, thinking about those qualities of the art making process which make it ideal for encouraging the kinds of sensitive and responsive interaction conditions highlighted above.

Engagement

An art therapy approach is ideal for enabling and encouraging infant-centred interactions as it draws both caregiver and baby into the process. Hall (2008) describes how infants were always interested in being involved in painting with their mothers and that the mothers responded with interest. The inclusion of art can quickly engage infants in play in what otherwise may be a strange environment for them. Art making can be seen as a very natural means of communication for young children, with creativity intrinsic within their play (Dissanayake, 2000; Bruce, 2005). Creative arts may also be a more authentic and effective way for many children to communicate without some of the restrictions imposed within verbal language (Duffy, 2010). The materials themselves, and the fact that infants are often seeing most of them for the first time, can encourage exploration. It's important that materials chosen are developmentally appropriate (Parashak, 2008), easy to grasp for small hands, and paper that can stand up to large gestural marks and lots of liquid so that the process is satisfying rather than frustrating to the infants.

Art making can also be engaging for the adults, encouraging them to play. Thought may be given to how the materials are presented in order to invite them in (Proulx, 2002; Armstrong and Howatson, 2015). Sometimes caregivers will not have made art as an adult, and likewise, it is often something outside of their domestic life. This can create the potential to do something different, to be imaginative, and to be playful together. Some caregivers may feel less stigma around a referral for support because art is involved and less anxiety about what they may be asked to do in the sessions with art as a focus. Goodman's research (2009) into the barriers to accessing support found caregivers reporting a preference for treatment in a non-mental health setting. Art therapy based in community settings or even within galleries may thus help sessions feel more accessible. The gallery setting has the added benefit of connecting families to a cultural resource which they may continue to access long after the art therapy intervention has ended.

Physical qualities

Attachment in the first months of life is primarily played out physically—the baby seeks physical proximity to their caregiver and later, as they start exploring, their physical availability. Interventions like Watch, Wait, and Wonder have highlighted that it is important to address this physicality of attachment relationships within therapeutic interactions rather than focusing solely on the caregiver's mental representations (Cohen et al., 1999). The use of art materials naturally introduces physicality into the therapy process. Caregiver and baby usually sit together, typically on the floor at the baby's level. There is a need for physical contact as caregivers support their babies to make art—they may help them to sit upright by holding them between their legs or support them to stand so they can dip their feet in paint (Hall, 2008; Armstrong and Howatson, 2015). There is also a prompt for pleasant physical touch from caregivers while cleaning up afterwards if baths are used at the end of sessions.

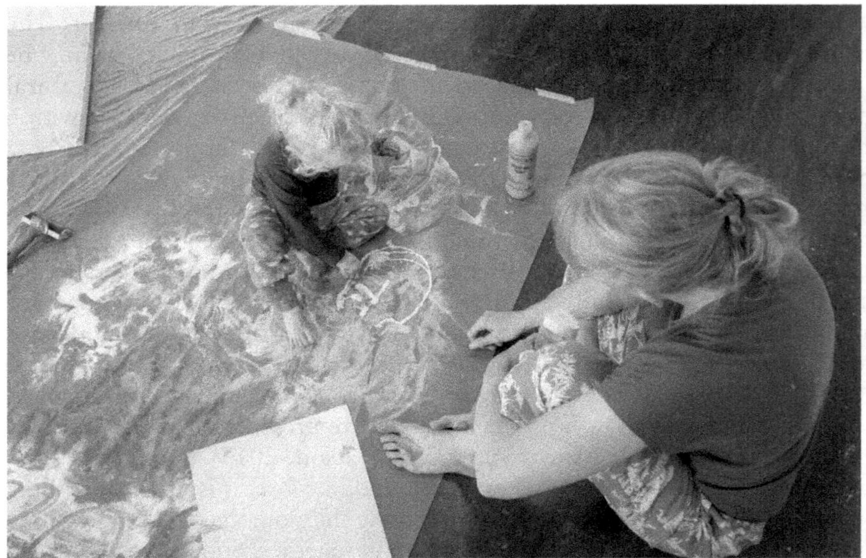

Figure 1.1 Infant and caregiver engaged in art making. Photograph by David P. Scott.

The materials also have their own physical qualities, which can add to the physicality and introduce positive sensory experiences. Paint, for example, may be smooth and slippery and give a pleasant physical sensation when babies slide it over the page or when their caregiver brushes it onto their feet. The brushes (or other painting tools like feathers or cotton balls) are soft, and caregivers can use them to respond with a gentle touch. Proulx (2002) describes how some materials' qualities may introduce specific symbolism, such as food or baby powder, which may also bring in associations with physical care. Bruce (2020) has described the importance that touch can take on in art psychotherapy, particularly where mothers' past traumas intrude into their present relationships with their infants (Figure 1.1).

Responsiveness and synchronous communication

Art making together, with encouragement to follow the baby's lead, can help to directly enhance responsiveness in the caregiver. Because the art materials are usually a novel sensation for the baby, with interesting tactile qualities, they generate plentiful displays of affect by the baby. These infant-initiated communications of affect give a wide range of affect expressions to which caregivers may tune in and respond. Affect expressions are sometimes spontaneously recognised by the caregivers or may initially need the art therapist to highlight them. This can be done by the art therapist directly reflecting them to the caregiver, by talking through the baby, or by modelling potential responses. Caregivers can be encouraged to reflect on the way infants respond to the materials. This allows them to practise attuning to their baby in a safe environment, and when the affect shown is safe—it is a response to the art as opposed to the caregiver themselves, which gives a safe distance.

The art therapist encourages caregivers to observe their babies and follow the interests they show in the materials. Art therapists have also described infant-led themes being naturally picked up by their whole group, allowing for the group as a whole to experience responsiveness (Lavey-Khan and Reddick, 2020). The art materials themselves can be a vehicle for the communication of affect through the way they are used and the colours chosen (Hosea, 2017). Even babies making art have a wide range of different qualities of marks, materials can be used in a hard or soft way, short or long marks, with stabbing motions or sweeping motions, they may start to make circular gestures. These convey babies' interest and are ripe for responding to. Even just by observing and maybe narrating what they see their baby try, a caregiver can practise attunement. It is also possible to offer an attuned response whilst staying within the art process, using the materials themselves as a way of offering attuned responses back (Armstrong and Howatson, 2015; Hosea, 2017). This can be modelled by the art therapist in the first instance and then picked up by the caregiver.

As the babies experience these positive responses in the context of a pleasant experience with the art materials, they will build positive associations to the art making and also to their parent. Caregivers interviewed about their experiences making art with their baby (Armstrong and Ross, 2022) described babies showing excitement when they got the art materials out which may be interpreted as a sign of positive anticipation. This suggests that the baby is demonstrating a positive association with the parent and the activity. This is important because having a positive association to their caregiver is a sign that the baby is internalising positive models of their interactions.

Caregivers also described babies turning to look at them, of looking together at the art making, of babies 'asking' them to join in, and of babies showing them the materials (Armstrong and Ross, 2021). These descriptions show babies being able to express their interest and then share it with their caregiver. Such descriptions demonstrate caregivers observing moments of intersubjectivity between them and their baby. They also described the ways in which they had responded by joining the baby and further that they had enjoyed these interactions themselves. These interactions show the potential within art making for interactional synchrony (Isabella and Belsky, 1991). Those caregivers were offering well timed responses, and the caregivers and babies were having two-way, mutually rewarding interactions. As we know from the literature above, these kinds of synchronous exchanges are fundamental in building strong attachment relationships (Svanberg, 1998). Therefore, if art making can be a vehicle to facilitate these synchronous exchanges, then there is encouraging potential for art to create change in the relationship.

Within a therapeutic setting, there may be increased opportunity for these moments of synchrony as the caregiver can focus fully on being present for the baby without the intrusions that may sometimes be present in domestic life. The art therapist may also model a way of being, which is sensitive to the baby and playful, and this may allow caregivers to also shift into a different mode of being with their baby. Art therapists are comfortable with 'not knowing,' which can be a useful stance towards infants to allow them to lead and leave space for what they communicate. If caregivers can adopt this stance, it allows them to be curious about their baby, be more receptive to their baby's approaches, and respond in a timely way which promotes synchrony.

Where both caregiver and baby are engaged in a shared piece of art making these exchanges often take on the rhythm of a serve-and-return communication themselves, each adding their mark then waiting to see the other's response. Arroyo and Fowler (2013) describe 'mirroring' between mothers and infants painting together in the way they used marks, colour, shape, and form. In a shared artwork, there is an acceptance of what the other has shared that parallels the caregiver's receptiveness and acceptance of the baby's affect. The added benefit here from using the medium of the art is that a visible record of this exchange is jointly created, and this artwork is something that can represent those moments of synchronicity.

Regulation

As discussed in the literature, caregivers can offer regulation to their baby during interactive exchanges. This may be through their presence when the baby is distressed or, as exchanges become more complex, a caregiver may be able to subtly shift affect through the use of slight 'deliberate missattunements' (Stern, 2000). Within the art process, it is inevitable that there will be some need for regulation. During a session, most babies will need to be soothed at some point to be 'up-regulated' to play or to be helped to contain when play becomes too chaotic. Parents are encouraged to offer this regulation using all the different channels available, especially through the art process itself.

Some materials may be able to promote regulation, and this can be modelled by the therapist. Proulx (2000) describes introducing shakers to a painting activity at the point an infant would lose their interest, thereby 'up-regulating' and prolonging their engagement. Where babies may be starting to feel dysregulated, the materials can contain too, for example, by offering absorbent paper if the paint is flowing off the page (Armstrong and Howatson, 2015) or by painting the inside of a box (Proulx, 2002). There is something very direct about these ways of offering regulation that may be more tangible to the caregiver, allowing them to practise with concrete ways to regulate that can then carry over into more subtle ways of communicating.

It is important to note here that the art therapist also provides regulation to the caregiver throughout. They offer containment so the materials don't become too messy and overwhelming so that they are able to remain engaged and playful. Hosea (2017) describes redirecting mess that is distressing a parent into something more positive when a baby spreading paint around the room on their feet is encouraged to make footprints on paper. In order to be best able to co-regulate their baby, caregivers need to feel well-regulated themselves (Rosanbalm and Murray, 2017). Taking part in the art process and using materials may be supporting this, with art engagement shown to aid regulation and increase positive mood valence (Fancourt et al., 2019). Caregivers making art with their babies have reported lowering of their own stress levels (Armstrong and Ross, 2022).

Agency and self-efficacy

I have spoken about how the qualities of mark making may be a vehicle for communication, but the process of mark making is also important to the babies' own development. When babies make a mark on the page, they see a direct result of their own actions—they feel their own agency. Matthews (1999) describes how early scribbles are not the result of accidental actions but intentional explorations on the part of the baby. He identifies different movements in mark making, e.g., sweeping, stabbing, and push-pull, that infants are investigating (Matthews, 1999). In exploring the impact they can make on the world, the baby builds their own sense of self-efficacy. This parallels their experiences of efficacy in their interactions, where they cry and a predictable response occurs. The tactile qualities of the materials and their feel upon the body may increase bodily awareness and their sense of themselves as an individual. Facilitating babies' self-efficacy is beneficial in its own right in terms of babies' own socio-emotional development; however, in the dyadic relationship it is also important in allowing caregivers to see their baby as an individual. Caregivers have identified changes they noticed during art making together, including those that represented agency, such as babies actively trying to make a line (Armstrong and Ross, 2022). By noticing these behaviours, we are seeing caregivers recognising their infant as an individual with their own sense of self, with whom they then have the potential to connect on an intersubjective level.

Reflective function

This connects to a caregiver's capacity for reflective function, which, as noted above, is related to strong attachments (Meins et al., 2002). In picking up these changes in their baby and consciously thinking about them, these caregivers demonstrated their capacity to reflect on their infant's mental states and intentions. As art making is a new experience for the infants, with textures and colours to explore, it prompts clear reactions from infants and may encourage parents to be curious about the infant's experience. Art therapists describe how this may allow caregivers to view their infant in a new way (Arroyo and Fowler, 2013; Hosea, 2017). Working to increase a parent's reflective capacity can be a successful intervention for attachment difficulties (Suchman et al., 2011). Caregivers can be directly encouraged to reflect during an art therapy session, and the art therapist can also 'think aloud' or model talking to the baby to draw attention to certain behaviours and to what the baby is experiencing or attempting. Within the structure of the session overall, there is usually time left at the end for the whole group to reflect (Armstrong and Ross, 2020). Some art therapists also create additional imagery of caregivers and babies together in photos or videos and caregivers can view these and reflect on the interactions (Hosea, 2017; Bruce, 2020).

Vignette—Mum and Caleb

Last week, Caleb had moved to the opposite side of the circle of painting dyads, at a distance from his mum. She had not moved towards him or sought to engage and eventually had stood up and walked towards the far side of the room. At this point, Caleb had approached Mum, and she swung him up over her head and then put him back down on his feet. He had moved away from her quickly back to the other side of the circle. We felt there was a fearfulness in his response and that, although intended as play, this had been too rough for him. As facilitators, we discussed ways they might be supported, and this week offered very large paper and trucks to dip in paint and roll. Caleb was interested by these and the textures he could see them making. Mum was more able to engage in this than in the previous week's painting and sat beside the big paper opposite him. Caleb rolled the truck to the art therapist, who rolled it back to him, following his lead in the game. She offered Mum a car to roll to Caleb, and they began a back-and-forth with the cars. The art therapist added some blobs of paint to the middle of the paper so the cars could be rolled through these and leave a track. Caleb sometimes chose to roll to Mum and sometimes to keep it in his hand through the paint.

Facilitators' notes

We had been surprised the week before by how rough Mum's play felt. Although intended playfully, it felt too much for a baby of Caleb's age, 13 months old, although robust and walking. We felt that his quick move away from Mum and lack of eye contact showed he had experienced this negatively. We wondered if Mum had felt excluded by his painting. It also seemed to us that Mum held an idea in her head of her baby that did not seem to match the real Caleb in front of her. She was missing cues and chances to engage, where he was receptive. In bringing the trucks in, we were hoping to meet both halfway to help them connect. The large paper and trucks connected with Mum's physicality and maybe also with some of her ideas about gender and what he should like. Caleb had been interested in paint and textures in previous weeks, so we thought this would also be engaging for him. In making tracks through the paint Caleb was seeing his own agency in the mark making, and so was Mum. She was getting to see him as a more active person in his own right, which opens up more potential for them to relate together. There is also safety in the back and forward with cars, allowing Caleb to negotiate the space between them and to approach and retreat from Mum within the game. We could also think about how this kind of play may parallel some of the 'serve and return' rhythms of early communication and maybe help Mum to respond to Caleb, where previously she seemed to find it hard if she was not the initiator. It was encouraging to see them finding ways to be together and to see positive moments of joint attention as they both looked at the vehicles and the resulting marks.

Conclusion

This chapter began with the World Health Organization's guidance that all young children should receive responsive care. In thinking about the kinds of interventions which may be useful in promoting that responsive care, they suggest that:

> They encourage and support sensitivity and responsiveness (care that is prompt, consistent, contingent, and appropriate to the child's cues, signals, behaviours and needs) or secure attachment. [They] ... improve caregivers' abilities to incorporate the child's signals and perspective ... facilitating the caregiver to be attuned to and identify the child's needs and wants, to follow the child's lead, help the child to focus, support the child's exploration and scaffold development. (WHO, 2020, p. 12)

This chapter has demonstrated the ways in which an art therapy approach answers this brief for a relationship intervention. Working towards responsive caregiving in the context of art therapy, we can draw on the qualities of the art process and art materials to facilitate sensitive and synchronous interactions. These responsive interactions may develop naturally as an integral part of the shared art process, or they may require more direct interventions from the art therapist to alert caregivers to their babies' signals.

They may also require therapeutic support from the art therapist to allow the caregiver to be sufficiently regulated themselves to be in a receptive state and to be able to follow their infant's lead. A benefit of having an art therapist facilitate art making for caregivers and their infants is that the art therapist can draw on their own art making knowledge and experience of the materials as a trained artist themselves but is also able to bring their therapeutic understanding of development and relationships when more support is needed. The art can be a hook that draws the caregiver and the baby together in shared activity and allows the therapeutic work to take place. We have seen how the baby experiences art making in ways that are about expressing, experimenting, and exploring, and how the art making can give the parent a new perspective on the baby's experience.

Art therapy has much to offer within perinatal and infant mental health services in a wide range of settings to create positive outcomes for children and their caregivers. It is hoped this approach can be incorporated into service structures and funding models. There is a need within research for further exploration of the mechanisms for changing interactions within the art therapy process, which we have suggested here, and how these might be demonstrated convincingly. For art therapy as a field, there is a need for more therapists to be trained to work dyadically and for encouragement to practitioners to work from the earliest ages where relationships are struggling.

References

Acquarone, S. (2004). *Infant-parent psychotherapy: A handbook*. London: Routledge.

All Party Parliamentary Group on Arts, Health and Wellbeing (APPGAHW) (2017). *Creative health inquiry report: The arts for health and wellbeing*, 2nd Edition. London: Creative Commons.

Ainsworth, M. S. (1989). Attachments beyond infancy. *American Psychologist*, 44(4), pp. 709–716.

Armstrong, V., Dalinkeviciute, E., and Ross, J. (2019). A dyadic art psychotherapy group for parents and infants – Piloting quantitative methodologies for evaluation. *International Journal of Art Therapy*, 24(3), pp. 113–124.

Armstrong, V. G. (2021). *Art therapy in a range of gallery-based arts interventions for the wellbeing of parents and infants*. University of Dundee: Royal Society for Public Health.

Armstrong, V. G., and Howatson, R. (2015). Parent-infant art psychotherapy: A creative dyadic approach to early intervention. *Infant Mental Health Journal*, 36(2), pp. 213–222.

Armstrong, V. G., and Ross, J. (2020). The evidence base for art therapy with parent and infant dyads: An integrative literature review. *International Journal of Art Therapy*, 25(3), pp. 103–118.

Armstrong, V. G., and Ross, J. (2021). Art boxes supporting parents and infants to share creative interactions at home: An art-based response to improve well-being during COVID-19 restrictions. *Public Health*, 193, pp. 109–112.

Armstrong, V. G., and Ross, J. (2022). The experiences of parents and infants using a home-based art intervention aimed at improving wellbeing and connectedness in their relationship. *Frontiers in Psychology*, 13, p. 732562. doi: 10.3389/fpsyg.2022.732562.

Arroyo, C., and Fowler, N. (2013). Before and after: A mother and infant painting group. *International Journal of Art Therapy*, 18(3), pp. 98–112.

Bakermans-Kranenburg, M. J., Van Ijzendoorn, M. H., and Juffer, F. (2003). Less is more: Meta-analyses of sensitivity and attachment interventions in early childhood. *Psychological Bulletin*, 129(2), pp. 195–215.

Ban, L., Gibson, J. E., West, J., Fiaschi, L., Oates, M. R., and Tata, L. J. (2012). Impact of socioeconomic deprivation on maternal perinatal mental illness presenting to UK general practice. *British Journal of General Practice*, 62(603), pp. 671–678.

Baradon, T. (2005). *The practice of psychoanalytic parent–infant psychotherapy: Claiming the baby*. Hove: Routledge.

Barlow, J., Schrader-McMillan, A., Axford, N., Wrigley, Z., Sonthalia, S., Wilkinson, T., Rawsthorn, M., Toft, A., and Coad, J. (2016). Review: Attachment and attachment-related outcomes in preschool children - a review of recent evidence. *Child and Adolescent Mental Health*, 21(1), pp. 11–20.

Bauer, A., Parsonage, M., Knapp, M., Iemmi, V., and Adelaja, B. (2014). *The cost of perinatal mental health problems*. London: Centre for Mental Health.

Belsky, J. (2001). Developmental risks (still) associated with early child care. *Journal of Child Psychology and Psychiatry*, 42(7), pp. 845–859.

Benoit, D. (2004). Infant-parent attachment: Definition, types, antecedents, measurement and outcome. *Paediatrics and Child Health*, 8(8), pp. 541–545.

Bergman, K., Sarkar, P., Glover, V., and O' Connor, T. G. (2010). Maternal prenatal cortisol and infant cognitive development: Moderation by infant-mother attachment. *Biological Psychiatry*, 67, pp. 1026–1032.

Bernier, A., Carlson, S. M., Deschenes, M., and Matte-Gagne, C. (2012). Social factors in the development of early executive functioning: A closer look at the caregiving environment. *Developmental Science*, 15(1), pp. 12–24.

Bigelow, A. E., MacLean, K., Proctor, J., Myatt, T., Gillis, R., and Power, M. (2010). Maternal sensitivity throughout infancy: Continuity and relation to attachment security. *Infant Behavior and Development*, 33(1), pp. 50–60.

Black, C., Ellis, M., and Harris L. (2015). Art, care and collaboration: The evaluation of Creative Families. *Making it together: An evaluative study of Creative Families an arts and mental health partnership between the South London Gallery and the Parental Mental Health Team*. London: King's Health PartnersAcademic, pp. 14–38.

Bowlby, J. (1997). *Attachment and loss, I: Attachment*. London: Pimlico.

Bruce, D. (2020). Cases on the border: Perinatal parent-infant work involving migrants, video analysis and art therapy. In S. Hogan (Ed), *Therapeutic arts in pregnancy, birth and new parenthood*. Routledge, pp. 228–242.

Bruce, D., and Hackett, S. S. (2020). Developing art therapy practice within perinatal parent-infant mental health. *International Journal of Art Therapy*, 26(3), pp. 111–122.

Bruce, T. (2005). Play, the universe and everything!. In J. Moyles (Ed), *The excellence of play*. Maidenhead: Open University Press, pp. 256–267.

Camoirano, A. (2017). Mentalizing makes parenting work: A review about parental reflective functioning and clinical interventions to improve it. *Frontiers in Psychology*, 8(1), pp. 1–12.

Cohen, N. J., Muir, E., Parker, C. J., *et al.* (1999). Watch, wait, and wonder: Testing the effectiveness of a new approach to mother-infant psychotherapy. *Infant Mental Health Journal*, 20(4), pp. 429–451.

Cummings, E. M., and Cicchetti, D. (1990). Toward a transactional model of relations between attachment and depression. In M. T. Greenberg, D. Cicchetti and E. M. Cummings (Eds), *Attachment in the preschool years: Theory, research, and intervention.* Chicago, United States: The University of Chicago Press, pp. 339–372.

De Wolff, M. S., and van Ijzendoorn, M. H. (1997). Sensitivity and attachment: A meta-analysis on parental antecedents of infant attachment. *Child Development*, 68(4), pp. 571–591.

Dissanayake, E. (2000). *Art and intimacy: How the arts began.* Seattle: University of Washington Press.

Duffy, B. (2010). Using creativity and creative learning to enrich the lives of young children at the Thomas Coran Centre. In C. Tims (Ed), *Born creative.* London: Demos, pp. 19–28.

Fancourt, D., Garnett, C., Spiro, N., West, R., and Mullensiefen, D. (2019). How do artistic creative activities regulate our emotions? Validation of the emotion regulation strategies for artistic creative activities scale (ERS-ACA). *PLoS One*, 14(2), pp. 1–22. doi:10.1371/journal.pone.0211362.

Fearon, R. P., Bakermans-Kranenburg, M. J., van Ijzendoorn, M. H., Lapsley, A., and Roisman, G. I. (2010). The significance of insecure attachment and disorganization in the development of children's externalizing behavior: A meta-analytic study. *Child Development*, 81(2), pp. 435–456.

Feldman, R. (2007). Parent – infant synchrony and the construction of shared timing; Physiological precursors, developmental outcomes, and risk conditions. *Journal of Child Psychology and Psychiatry and Allied Disciplines*, 4(3–4), pp. 329–354.

Field, T. (2018). Postnatal anxiety prevalence, predictors and effects on development: A narrative review. *Infant Behavior and Development*, 51, pp. 24–32.

Fonagy, P., Sleed, M., and Baradon, T. (2016). Randomized controlled trial of parent-infant psychotherapy and treatment as usual for parents with mental health problems and young infants. *Infant Mental Health Journal*, 37(2), pp. 97–114.

Goodman, J. H. (2009). Women's attitudes, preferences, and perceived barriers to treatment for perinatal depression. *Birth*, 36(1), pp. 60–69.

Grace, S. L., Evindar, A., and Stewart, D. E. (2003). The effect of postpartum depression on child cognitive development and behavior: A review and critical analysis of the literature. *Archives of Women's Mental Health*, 6(4), pp. 263–274.

Granat, A., Gadassi, R., Gilboa-Schechtman, E., and Feldman, R. (2017). Maternal depression and anxiety, social synchrony, and infant regulation of negative and positive emotions. *Emotion*, 17(1), pp. 11–27.

Habib, C. (2012). Paternal perinatal depression: An overview and suggestions towards an intervention model. *Journal of Family Studies*, 18(1), pp. 4–16.

Hall, P. (2008). Painting together: An art therapy approach to mother-infant relationships. In Case C. and Dalley T. (Eds), *Art therapy with children: From infancy to adolescence.* New York: Routledge/Taylor and Francis Group, pp. 20–35.

Harrison, S. E., Ayers, S., Quigley, M. A., Stein, A., and Alderdice, F. (2021). Prevalence and factors associated with postpartum posttraumatic stress in a population-based maternity survey in England. *Journal of Affective Disorders*, 279, pp. 749–756.

Hibbins, A., and Turner, L. (2020). Culture is for babies, gathering of strangers: *Civic engagement and education at the Whitworth*. Available at: https://civicengagementandeducation.wordpress.com/2020/11/12/culture-is-for-babies/ (Accessed: 16 September 2021).

Hogan, S. (2015). Mothers making art: Using participatory art to explore the transition to motherhood. *Journal of Applied Arts and Health*, 6(1), pp. 23–32.

Hosea, H. (2017). Amazing Mess: Mothers get in touch with their infants through the vitality of painting together. In J. Meyerowitz-Katz and D. Reddick (Eds), *Art therapy in the early years: Therapeutic interventions with infants, toddlers and their families*. London: Routledge, pp. 104–117.

Isabella, R. A., and Belsky, J. (1991). Interactional synchrony and the origins of infant-mother attachment: A replication study. *Child Development*, 62(2), pp. 373–384.

Johansson, M., Benderix, Y., and Svensson, I. (2020). Mothers' and fathers' lived experiences of postpartum depression and parental stress after childbirth: A qualitative study. *International Journal of Qualitative Studies on Health and Well-being*, 15(1), 1722564. doi:10.1080/17482631.2020.1722564.

Jones, A. (2006). How video can bring to view pathological defensive processes and facilitate the creation of triangular space in perinatal parent–infant psychotherapy. *Infant Observation*, 9(2), pp. 109–123.

Kingston, D., and Tough, S. (2014). Prenatal and postnatal maternal mental health and school-age child development: A systematic review. *Maternal and Child Health Journal*, 18(7), pp. 1728–1741.

Klawetter, S., and Frankel, K. (2018). Infant mental health: A lens for maternal and child mental health disparities. *Journal of Human Behavior in the Social Environment*, 28(5), 557–569. doi:10.1080/10911359.2018.1437495

Lavey-Khan, S., and Reddick, D. (2020). The arts in psychotherapy painting together: A parent-child dyadic art therapy group. *The Arts in Psychotherapy*, 70 (September). doi:10.1016/j.aip.2020.101687

Maternal Mental Health Alliance (2020). *Map of specialist community perinatal mental health teams (UK)*. London: Maternal Mental Health Alliance.

Matthews, J. (1999). *The art of childhood and adolescence: The construction of meaning*. London: Falmer.

Meins, E., Fernyhough, C., Wainwright, R., Das Gupta, M., Fradley, E., and Tuckey, M. (2002). Maternal mind-mindedness and attachment security as predictors of theory of mind understanding. *Child Development*, 73(6), pp. 1715–1726.

Meyerowitz-Katz, J. (2017). The crisis of the cream cakes: An infants food refusal as a representation of intergenerational trauma. In Julia Meyerowitz-Katz and D. Reddick (Eds), *Art therapy in the early years: Therapeutic interventions with infants, toddlers and their families*. London: Routledge, pp. 118–132.

Mikulincer, M., Shaver, P. R., Gillath, O., and Nitzberg, R. A. (2005). Attachment, caregiving, and altruism: Boosting attachment security increases compassion and helping. *Journal of Personality and Social Psychology*, 89, 817–839. doi:10.1037/0022-3514.89.5.817

Moullin, S., Waldfogel, J., and Washbrook, E. (2014). *Baby bonds: Parenting, attachment and a secure base for children*. London: Sutton Trust (England).

Murray, A. D., and Yingling, J. L. (2000). Competence in language at 24 months: Relations with attachment security and home stimulation. *The Journal of Genetic Psychology*, 161(2), pp. 133–140.

Murray, L., Fiori-Cowley, A., Hooper, R., and Cooper, P. (1996). The impact of postnatal depression and associated adversity on early mother-infant interactions and later infant outcome. *Child Development*, 67(5), pp. 2512–2526.

Music, G. (2011). Trauma, helpfulness and selfishness: The effect of abuse and neglect on altruistic, moral and pro-social capacities. *Journal of Child Psychotherapy*, 37(2), pp. 113–128.

Newton, K., Taylor Buck, E., Weich, S., and Uttley, L. (2022). A review and analysis of the components of potentially effective perinatal mental health interventions for infant development and mother-infant relationship outcomes, *Development and Psychopathology*, 24, pp. 37–54.

O'Hara, M. W., and Wisner, K. L. (2014). Perinatal mental illness: Definition, description and aetiology Michael. *Best Practice and Research Clinical Obstetrics and Gynaecology*, 28(1), pp. 3–12.

Parashak, S. T. (2008). Object relations and attachment theory: Creativity of mother and child in the single parent family. In Christine Kerr and J. Hoshino (Eds), *Family art therapy: Foundations of theory and practice*. London: Routledge, pp. 65–93.

Perry, C., Thurston, M., and Osborn, T. (2008). Time for me: The arts as therapy in postnatal depression. *Complementary therapies in clinical practice*, 14(1), pp. 38–45.

Proulx, L. (2000). Container, contained, containment. *Canadian Art Therapy Association Journal*, 14(1), pp. 3–6.

Proulx, L. (2002). Strengthening ties, parent-child-dyad: Group art therapy with toddlers and parents. *American Journal of Art Therapy*, 40(4), pp. 238–258.

Rayment, A. (2017). Side by side: An early years' art therapy group with a parallel therapeutic parent support group. In Julia Meyerowitz-Katz and D. Reddick (Eds), *Art therapy in the early years: Therapeutic interventions with infants, toddlers and their families*. London and New York: Routledge, pp. 165–177.

Rosanbalm, K., and Murray, D. W. (2017). *Caregiver co-regulation across development: A practice brief. OPRE Brief #2017-80*. Washington: Office of Planning, Research and Evaluation, Administration for Children and Families, US. Department of Health and Human Services.

Schore, A. N. (2001). Effects of a secure attachment relationship on right brain development, affect regulation, and infant mental health. *Infant Mental Health Journal*, 22, pp. 7–66.

Shonkoff, J. P., Garner, A. S., and Committee on psychosocial aspects of child and family health, Committee on early childhood adoption and dependent care, and Section on developmental and behavioural pediatrics (2012). The lifelong effects of early childhood adversity and toxic stress. *Pediatrics*, 129(1), pp. 232–236.

Sroufe, L. A. (2005). Attachment and development: A prospective, longitudinal study from birth to adulthood. *Attachment and Human Development*, 7(4), pp. 349–367.

Steele, H., Steele, M., and Fonagy, P. (1996). Associations among attachment classifications of mothers, fathers and their infants. *Child Development*, 67(2), pp. 541–555.

Stern, D. N. (2000). *The interpersonal world of the infant: A view from psychoanalysis and developmental psychology*. New York: Basic Books.

Suchman, N. E., DeCoste, C., Castiglioni, N., McMahon, T. J., Rounsaville, B., and Mayes, L. (2011). The Mothers and Toddlers program, an attachment-based parenting intervention for substance-using women: Results at 6-week follow-up in a randomized clinical pilot. *Infant Mental Health Journal*, 32(4), pp. 427–449.

Svanberg, P. O. G. (1998). Attachment, resilience and prevention. *Journal of Mental Health*, 7(6), pp. 543–578.

Trevarthen, C. (2001). Intrinsic motives for companionship in understanding: Their origin, development and significance for infant mental health. *Infant Mental Health Journal*, 22(1–2), pp. 95–131.

Tronick, E. (2007). *The neurobehavioral and social-emotional development of infants and children*. New York: Norton.

Van Der Voort, A., Juffer, F., and Bakermans-Kranenburg, M. J. (2014). Sensitive parenting is the foundation for secure attachment relationships and positive social-emotional development of children. *Journal of Children's Services*, 9(2), pp. 165–176.

Williams, M. (2020). *Fathers reaching out - Why dads matter*: Available at: https://dadmatters.org.uk/fathers-reaching-out-why-dads-matter/ (Accessed: 16 September 2021).

Winberg, J. (2005). Mother and newborn baby: Mutual regulation of physiology and behavior— A selective review. *Developmental Psychobiology*, 47, pp. 217–229.

World Health Organization (2020). *Improving early childhood development: WHO guideline*.

Xeros-Constantinides, S., Boland, B., and Bishop, L. (2017). Journeying to Connect: Promoting post-natal healing and relationship formation through the CONNECT Group Art-Therapy Program for distressed mothers and infants: A clinical practice article. *Australian Journal of Child and Family Health Nursing*, 14(2), pp. 4–11.

Chapter 2

Community music therapy with refugee children in transit camps on the Greek island of Chios

'Like one family, together'

Mitsi Akoyunoglou and Giorgos Tsiris

Chios, 2020, Mitsi's fieldnotes

During a focus group discussion following a three-month period of music therapy groups, a teenage participant said, "we were like one family, together," and another one added, "the music does not mind if one is from Algeria, the other one from another country ... all of us we were one country." These music therapy groups took place with unaccompanied minors residing at the Registration and Identification Centre for refugees on the Greek island of Chios. Despite their limited English, the participants articulated their experiences vividly at the end of music therapy. While reading the focus group transcript, I paused to reflect on the multiple areas of impact the various groups I facilitated had on the lives of refugee children who lived temporarily on the island in numerous different contexts.

The so-called 'refugee crisis' began in 2015, when Chios, among other Greek islands, became the first port of entry to Europe. This crisis soon arrived right outside my door, and I felt an urge to respond. As someone living on the island for more than 25 years, I wanted to act as a citizen first, then as an activist. In tandem, I began offering my voluntary services as a professional music therapist. Over the next five years, I saw the music therapy groups changing and transforming in line with the changing needs of the children, their communities, and the wider socio-political landscape. Due to changes in Greek and European policies, refugees' length of stay on the island differed from year to year. Starting in June 2015, refugees would stay only for three or four days before moving to a different setting in another part of Greece. A year later, they would stay in Chios' transit camps for a couple of months, while others who arrived even later were obliged to stay for more than a year, or even two, waiting for the processing of their asylum papers.

I remember the first music therapy group, which took place at the detention centre for refugees in the area of Mersinidi. I was shocked to see so many people, mainly families with young children, given space to sleep outside the village's cemetery. With the support of some friends, I facilitated the first group.

DOI: 10.4324/9781003265610-3

After placing a large tarpaulin for all to sit on, we distributed coloured markers and paper sheets for the children to draw. Around 40 children gathered, grabbed a couple of markers each and started drawing. Houses, birds, butterflies, flowers, trees, and boats started appearing. As the children completed their drawings, I improvised a hello song while playing the autoharp,[1] and I witnessed music's power in action once again; children did not speak the same language and did not know each other, yet they became a group, singing and moving together. They participated in call and response, and action songs with great enthusiasm. The unfamiliar and hostile environment of the informal camp was transformed. My friends and I left about two hours later with a promise to return. Indeed, this was the beginning of a five-year journey offering community music therapy to refugee children in Chios on a weekly basis.

Points of departure

The difficult and adverse conditions that accompany the involuntary dislocation of refugees impact refugee children's physical and psychological health negatively (Betancourt et al., 2019; Hodes, 2019; Hodes and Vostanis, 2019; Yayan et al., 2020; Papadopoulos, 2021). The refugee experience holds many diverse challenges, and even though children are commonly considered as being resilient, psychosocial support can be of the essence (Kuriansky, 2019).

Overall, there is limited research pertaining to music therapy in refugee camps (Storsve et al., 2010; Mallon and Antink, 2021; Parker et al., 2021) and an even greater sparsity of literature focusing on transit refugee camps. In this chapter, we aspire to contribute practice-led knowledge to this area of work. Through a process-driven—rather than outcomes-oriented—approach, we explore community music therapy with refugee children in various camp settings on the Greek island of Chios (Figure 2.1).

Our narrative adopts an auto-ethnographically informed stance (Poulos, 2021) and is based on the experience of the first author (Mitsi), who has worked as the music therapist in this context. Our writing offers an overview of four key phases of the community music therapy journey with refugee children in various transit camps. It is enriched with in-depth accounts and vignettes. These vignettes, drawn and compiled from fieldnotes kept by the first author and diaries kept by a small group of volunteer educators, are used to provide rich descriptions of the settings, the unique circumstances, and the various music therapy practices. An ongoing critical discussion between the two authors (Mitsi and Giorgos) allowed for the reflexive interpretation and articulation of these narratives presented below. Our respective positionings as white, middle-class individuals originating from Greece and trained as music therapists in the US and UK respectively coloured our perspectives and understandings.

As the reader engages with this chapter, we invite them to keep the following in mind:

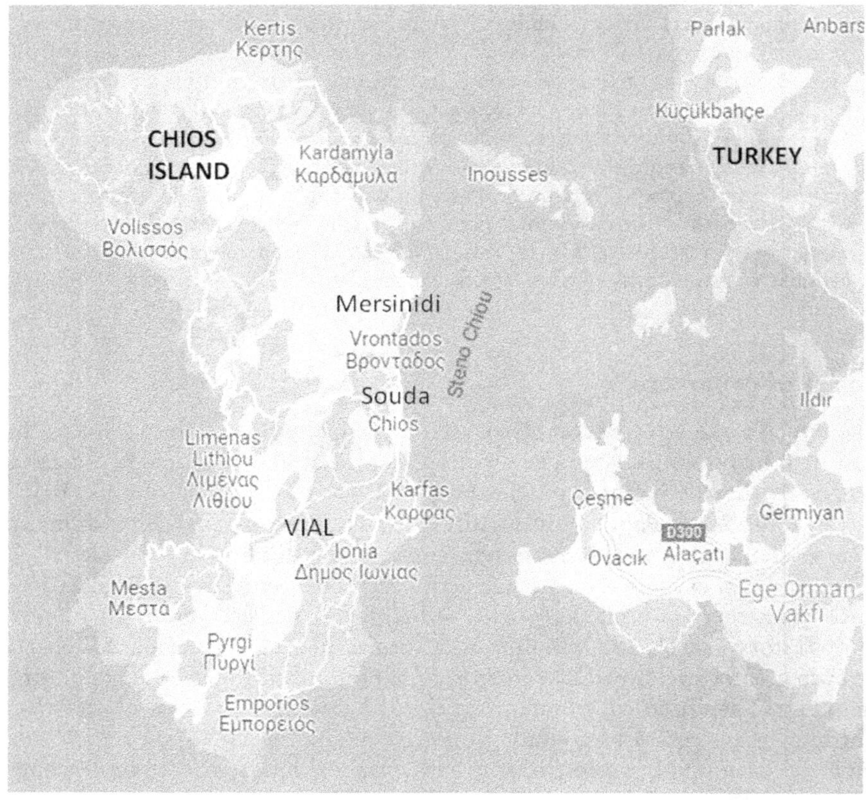

Figure 2.1 Chios Island, Greece, with marked locations of transit camps Mersinidi, Souda, and the Registration and Identification Centre of Chios (VIAL). Image from Google Maps (Map of Chios Island, Greece, 2022).

Firstly, we use the term 'refugee' for simplicity throughout the chapter to refer to all children and adolescents living in transit camps. However, we do not assume refugees as being a homogeneous group of people. It would perhaps be appropriate to consider people on the move as being 'persons of concern,' a term that encompasses immigrants, refugees, asylum seekers, displaced, and stateless people (Crisp, 2009). In any case, it should be clarified that each person's identity as a refugee is interlinked to their unique sociocultural and political conditions and does not imply or assume any mental or other health predicaments.

Secondly, again for simplicity, we use the term 'children' to refer to all young people who participated in music therapy. At times, different groups were addressed to young children, unaccompanied minors, or adolescents.

We would also like to stress some basic ethical considerations for music therapists who may work with refugee children residing in transit camps: (a) the basic survival needs of children should be cared for first (e.g., when a child is hungry, you ensure food is provided), (b) professionalism, consistency and diligence should be offered even when one is volunteering (e.g., regularity and consistency of groups should be maintained), and (c) the music therapist should be driven by a deep respect for equality, diversity, inclusion, and belonging (e.g., all children are welcome, and they participate of their own free will).

Journey phase 1

In June 2015, the detention centre for refugees in Mersinidi was overcrowded, with many young children living in dire conditions. That month, on a Saturday morning, the first music therapy group took place and was the first of many groups to follow.

The music therapy groups were open to all refugee children and were organised once or twice a week depending on the weather conditions, as sessions were taking place outdoors within the camps. Since then, and for the next five years, music therapy groups have been organised in all informal and formal refugee camps in Chios.

During the summer of 2015, partly due to the unpreparedness of the municipality to receive and host large numbers of refugees, informal camps were formed, funded, and run mainly by volunteers. As a result, lots of small camping tents were set up to accommodate refugees during their stay in Chios (Figure 2.2). The United Nations High Commissioner for Refugees (UNHCR) began collaborating with the local authorities in September 2015, and since then, formal camps have begun operating first in Souda and then in VIAL (that is, the Registration and Identification Centre of Chios).

Vignette 1 (Municipal Garden, October 2015, Mitsi's fieldnotes)

In the first four months, we ran groups once, twice, or even three times a week—depending on the number of children and their needs—at the informal camp that was set up at the Municipal Garden of Chios town. This was a self-organised camp, functioning with the help of a small group of volunteers from the island. In September 2015, the UNHCR came to the island to oversee the living conditions of the refugees, and in October, Psychological First Aid training was offered to those working with refugees. This training brought a different perspective to how I approached the music therapy groups and changed the focus of the groups: I concentrated on enhancing feelings of safety, fostering togetherness, connecting children through communal active music participation, and strengthening their voice (literally and metaphorically) through singing.

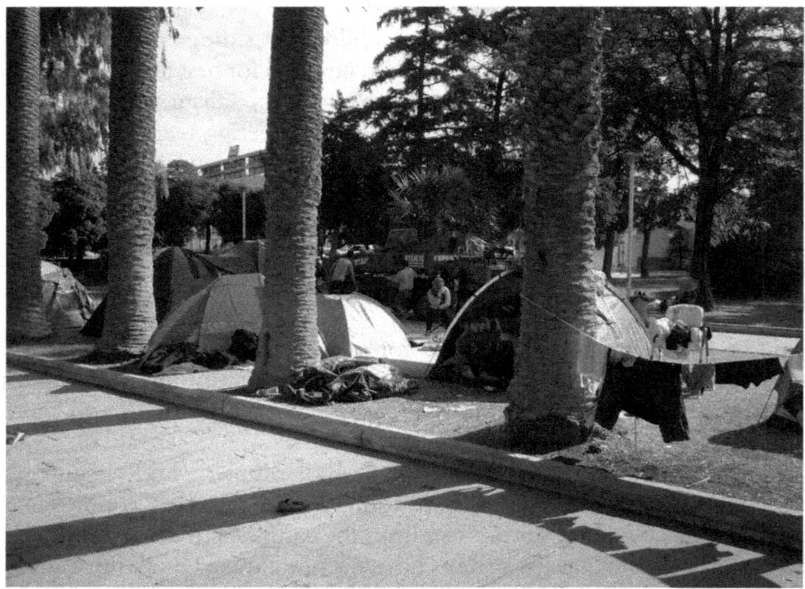

Figure 2.2 Small tents put up within the Municipal Garden. Photograph by Vassilis Pahoundakis.

Setting the scene: Then and now

That summer was characterised as 'the long summer of migration,' and 2015 as the year of the European humanitarian refugee crisis. Greece has been one of the countries of entry to Europe, and thousands of refugees have been crossing to Europe via the North Aegean Islands. Specifically, Chios, due to its proximity to the Turkish shoreline, has become a first port of entry for many refugees fleeing from their homeland due to war and wider socio-political and economic issues over the last years. The Chios strait is only three nautical miles, and refugees—often from Iraq, Syria, and Afghanistan—arrive on the island in small, yet crowded dinghies despite the dangers, hoping to reach a European destination.

During the second half of 2015, more than 100,000 people came through Chios; twice the population of the island. It is evident from the UNHCR data that the numbers decreased when, in March 2016, the European Union and Turkey reached an agreement (Council of the EU PRESS, 2016) that aimed at stopping the flow of migration, and refugees were halted from migrating without control to other European countries (UNHCR, 2017). To comprehend the differences in numbers, during the month of December 2015, more than 21,000 refugees arrived in Chios, and in December 2016, only 421.

In 2016, following the 'hotspot' approach,[2] the Registration and Identification Centre of Chios—called 'VIAL'—was established with a capacity to house about 1,100 refugees (Global Detention Project, 2019). VIAL was a former aluminium waste processing factory. To enter the camp, you needed permission from UNHCR, the International Organization for Migration (IOM) or some other non-governmental organisation (NGO), the Greek Ministry of Migration and Asylum, the police, and the administration of the camp. When one did not work at the camp and wished to visit the camp as a volunteer once or twice a week for only a couple of hours at a time, then additional permissions needed to be cleared.

Since 2015 the situation of refugee camps on the island has been changing radically. These changes required several adjustments for the music therapy groups to happen and provided opportunities for Mitsi to run diverse groups with refugee children in these settings.

Journey phase 2

Within the first few months following the summer of 2015, the music therapy groups began adopting a specific format. The groups were open to all children, from 2 to 14 years old, and were one-off gatherings since the duration of people's stay on the island was typically about three to four days. The following composite vignettes present and describe the issues faced, challenges tackled, and the way the groups were implemented at the informal, self-organised camps.

Vignette 2 (Municipal Garden, September 28, 2015, compilation from Mitsi's fieldnotes and two volunteers' diaries)

One of the main issues was where to set up our tarpaulins so that there would be enough space for children to gather, draw, sing, move, and play. The Municipal Garden was full of tents. Not much space was available for the gathering. We were a group of six volunteers that afternoon: four educators, a music teacher, and a music therapist. After a short exploratory walk around the area, to get an estimate of the number of children and to locate a place to anchor, we chose to set up on the opposite side from where we usually sat. We placed two 4 by 5 metres tarpaulins, taped two 4-metre-long sheets of paper, and spread many coloured markers.

Only a few children gathered in the beginning, but after a little while, we counted more than 30. Along with the children, some mothers came and sat in the circle. Four older teenagers, travelling together, drew sketches of each other's faces. When Mitsi took the autoharp out of its case and started singing, children turned towards her, sat up straight, left the markers on the papers, and changed places in order to come closer to her (Figure 2.3). Gradually they began singing along. We first greeted them with a hello song and then moved to call-and-response songs from Morocco and Ghana, such as *Ram Sam Sam* and *Che Che Kule*. We made shakers from toilet rolls and balloons. Then, we stood up and formed a big circle. Singing, playing, and moving reinforced the formation of one big group. Everyone coordinated their movements, kept the rhythm, and sang. The group lasted for about two hours.

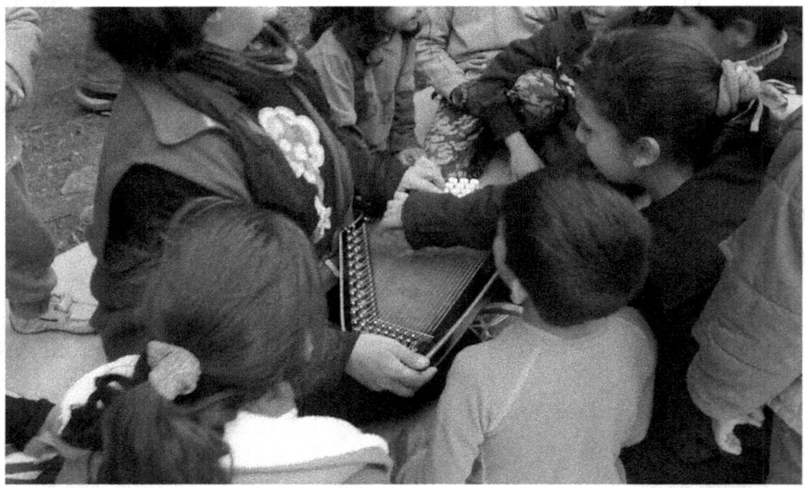

Figure 2.3 Group at the Municipal Garden. Photograph by Vicky Georgouli.

Vignette 3 (Chios Municipal Garden, October 5, 2015, compilation from Mitsi's fieldnotes and a volunteer's diary)

This was a very different afternoon. There seemed to be tension among the children; most had arrived on that day after a difficult journey—small inflatable boats, overcrowded, with windy conditions. Some children approached, took a couple of markers, and left. Some drew on other children's drawings, while others collected markers and refused to share with the group. Stress, difficulty in collaborating, and lack of attention were evident in all children. The group included youngsters from many different countries (Syria, Afghanistan, Palestine, Iraq, and more), and a young girl with Down syndrome joined the group as well. Once the music began, children started participating in a more inclusive manner. At the beginning some sang, others kept the rhythm with their bodies, and others seemed attentive but not actively participating. After demonstrating how to make a shaker, all children engaged in making their own. With the shakers at hand, many rhythm games kept the music going and, after a while, everyone in the circle began to sing in unison with louder voices. At the end, a girl from Syria with big blue eyes approached and said in English, 'thank you for making us smile.' Her face is unforgettable.

Each group and each session was unique. The space changed every time, and the number of children fluctuated from very few up to 90. The group energy differed depending partly on when the children had arrived on the island. Their engagement with the group was determined by their sense of emotional, psychological, and physiological wellbeing. The number and composition of volunteers depended each time on people's availability, and the activities were adapted to each group's needs. All these unpredictable and fluid factors required a flexible approach allowing for the unexpected.

Theoretical reflections: Children in a transit refugee camp

The life of refugees from the time of 'flight' from homeland to resettlement in a new host environment has been characterised by Reyes (1999) as 'an extreme case of decontextualization and recontextualization' (p. 16). There is an ongoing discussion in the literature about refugee children's adaptation skills and natural resilience that act as protective factors in relation to life stressors and context vulnerability that can act as risk factors (Daud et al., 2008; Papadopoulos, 2018; Weissbecker et al., 2019; Motti-Stefanidi et al., 2020).

Refugee children who are living temporarily either in detention centres or transit refugee camps face, to varying degrees, a range of psychosocial, emotional, and cultural challenges. Even though each child would handle such difficulties differently, prolonged exposure to adversities might compromise children's health and their physical, mental, emotional, and social growth (Vaghri et al., 2019). Refugee children might experience pre-flight phase stress (related, for example, to war, dislocation from home, loss of family members or friends), flight phase stress (related, for example, to poverty, hunger, deprivation of education, violence and exploitation) as well as resettlement phase stress. The latter might be related, for example, to family housing or financial difficulties, loss of community support, and acculturation stress as refugee children try to adjust to and integrate in a new culture, including language barriers, adaptation to a new school environment, and isolation stress as minority groups in the host country (Motti-Stefanidi et al., 2020). However, these stressors do not necessarily lead to the development of pathological stress or mental disorders in children (Daud et al., 2008; Vaghri et al., 2019).

Although children are resilient and can often cope with difficult experiences in healthy and productive ways, experience of traumatic events can trigger somatic symptoms, such as stomach aches, headaches, or other pain, that do not seem to have a physical cause. Children might exhibit anxiety, sadness, edginess, or sleeping problems. They may have trouble paying attention, lack a desire to play or engage in activities, and might be preoccupied with persistent thoughts or emotions often pertaining to past traumatic experiences (Fox, 2002; Cheng and Zarinnegar, 2020; Motti-Stefanidi et al., 2020). As Papadopoulos (2002) notes, when working with refugee children, one needs to remain aware not only of the vulnerability, disorientation, and pain that children may experience but also of their inherent resilience. Vulnerability, on the one hand, can be the result of four main factors: the living conditions, the underlying conditions, the triggering conditions, and the environmental conditions (Papadopoulos, 2019). Resilience, on the other hand, is based on three factors: the child's personality dispositions, their supportive family environment, and an external support system 'that encourages and reinforces the child's efforts to cope and instil in the child positive values' (Daud et al., 2008, p. 2).

The Psychological First Aid (PFA) steps are *listen*, *protect*, and *connect*, and PFA aims to attend to five basic principles: safety, calmness, connectedness, self and community efficacy, and hope (Dieltjens et al., 2014; Wang et al., 2021). In this context of work, PFA focuses on reducing distress. It improves functioning and coping, enhances safety and comfort, and establishes non-obtrusive and compassionate human connection. PFA can calm survivors who may be overwhelmed, agitated, and distraught. It can connect neighbours and other refugee children within the camp. It provides emotional support through sharing in activities and experiences of connectedness, safety, and group strength. Although literature seems to support the benefits of its use and various PFA interventions have been identified, there seems to be a lack of empirical evidence regarding its effectiveness (Shultz and Forbes, 2013; Dieltjens et al., 2014; Wang et al., 2021). This does not necessarily limit PFA's impact, which is practically evident in the humanitarian field by its widely used principles as an early intervention, but future rigorous research is needed.

As noted previously, children's natural resilience can play an important and protective role, but trauma, extreme stress, and anxiety can interfere with their learning and wellbeing. This reality constitutes caring for and supporting the wellbeing of refugee children crucial for their healthy development, especially during their stay in transit camps. Having as a starting point the PFA principles, a community music therapy approach for psychosocial support was designed, implemented, evaluated, and revised accordingly in order to meet the needs of the children.

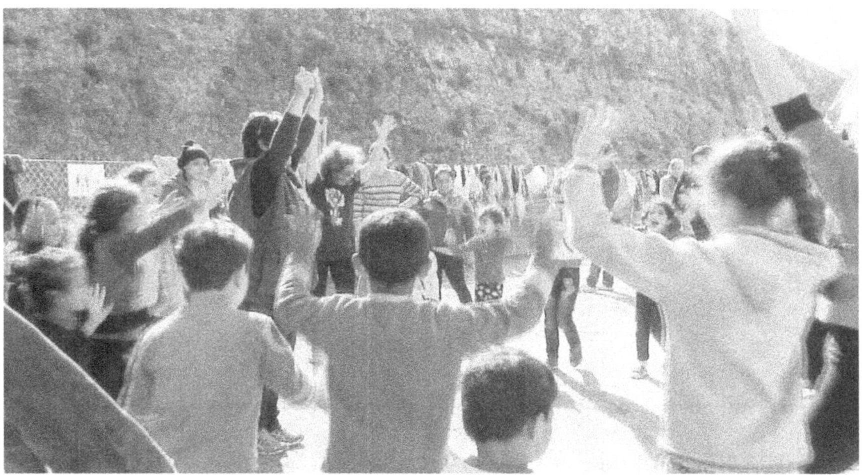

Figure 2.4 Large group at Souda Camp. Photograph by Vicky Georgouli.

Journey phase 3

Once the self-organised camp in the Municipal Garden closed, people were moved to a more organised camp which was operated by local authorities and UNHCR in Souda; an area close to the centre of Chios town. Refugees began to stay for a longer period of time—more than a month or two—and children participated in a number of music therapy groups. This allowed Mitsi to design and implement community-oriented music activities that were also guided by trauma-informed related approaches (Heiderscheit and Murphy, 2021). The groups always took place outdoors, so in the wintertime groups were organised once a week weather permitting (Figure 2.4).

Vignette 4 (Souda, January 9, 2016, compilation from Mitsi's fieldnotes and a volunteer's diary)

This Saturday the weather was nice. It was sunny, and we were able to go to Souda. Eighteen children gathered. They were drawing for about an hour, being very attentive and concentrated, and a small number of adults joined as well, mostly women. We have learned some words in Arabic, and we are able to communicate with them better. We conversed with a young lady who had a daughter and five sisters. They were all travelling with their mother to reach their final destination, Norway. She told us that she had another five siblings, a total of 11 brothers and sisters, yet one sister and one brother were killed during the war in Syria. While narrating her story, she seemed well composed and emotionally restrained.

The hello song captured children's attention right away. All children came to play the autoharp and accompany the song, while Mitsi was changing the chords. We sang four call-and-response songs and accompanied these with body percussion motives. The children, while singing, were trying to remember the rhythmic motives, to keep a steady beat, and to maintain eye contact with the music therapist. We had formed a standing circle and for the last song, we opened a coloured parachute. Initially, the children had difficulty keeping a common pulse with the parachute movements, but along with the songs, after a while, their movements were coordinated and unified. At the end, all group members wanted to know when we would be back again. Now that they stay a little longer in the camp, we are able to meet them again next time we visit.

In 2017, the situation shifted radically. Socio-political changes on a European, but also on a national and local level, pressed for a different approach. People from the local society began to express their objection against the hotspot and the prolonged stay of refugees, and the emotional and psychological atmosphere surrounding refugees became more difficult. This resulted in stricter procedures, and a number of permits had to be secured in order for the music therapy groups to continue. Fortunately, authorities were positively positioned, and we were able to obtain authorisation from the director of the camp, the police, as well as the Ministry of Education and Religious Affairs. The groups for the children continued, but less frequently, partly due to the overcrowded conditions of the camp making it difficult to identify a space to set up.

Vignette 5 (VIAL, November 25, 2017, compilation from Mitsi's fieldnotes and two volunteers' diaries)

The number of refugees residing in VIAL has increased a lot; the tents are growing in numbers, and not much space is available for our group to set up. Also, the access conditions are changing. We are now obliged to obtain permission to the hotspot.

Today, we went first to the camp's police so that they could designate the area where we could place our tarpaulins and we also met the camp's director. We set up where they told us; in the middle of a dirt road that was muddy due to rain in previous days. About 60 children gathered and quickly the tarpaulin got dirty and uninviting to draw. As soon as the music began, children became more open, their voices were tuned to the singing, and they joined the group. A while later, the police came to check on us. This was the first time that we felt observed in the groups by authorities and we experienced issues of trust.

The camp is becoming more difficult to enter, there are more restrictions for both refugees and volunteers, and only NGO employees have permits. Now that refugees are obliged to stay on the island for longer periods of time waiting for their asylum papers to be processed, it is even more vital to provide community-based groups for psychosocial support of children. This time, the official Registration and Identification Camp, VIAL, presented several difficulties that were new to us. From now on we need to secure permission to run the groups and also get validated from the Ministry of Education and Religious Affairs.

Theoretical reflections: Music therapy, crisis, adversity

Music therapists have been providing support in response to various humanitarian crises around the globe (Gonzalez et al., 2020). Over the last decade, numerous music therapy projects and music-based methods have focused on supporting the health and quality of life of refugees. It is well documented that the non-verbal and creative nature of music making facilitates emotional expression and reduces isolation (Bensimon et al., 2008; Garrido et al., 2015; Sutton, 2002). Culture-centred as well as community music therapy can provide refugees with an environment that promotes a sense of wellbeing and social inclusion (Enge, 2015) and enhances 'their ability to function as healthy members of society' (Abdulbaki and Berger, 2020, p. 10). As documented in the literature, music therapy interventions have focused on providing refugees with a non-verbal form of communication, helping reduce anxiety levels, regaining self-trust and feelings of self-efficacy, as well as promoting integration with the transit or host country and strengthen social interaction (Enge, 2015; Garrido et al., 2015; Akoyunoglou, 2019). Studies on music therapy and trauma survivors suggest that group music improvisation, composition, and songwriting can offer an avenue for expressing emotions, building confidence, strengthening group cohesion, sharing experiences of loss, and ultimately creating secure bonds between people (Choi, 2010; Davis, 2010; McFerran and Teggelove, 2011; Enge, 2015).

The refugee experience can hold many stressors. It has often been viewed through a sociocultural lens and described as a potentially traumatic event in terms of development, and identity. Published practice and research accounts with refugees focus on a variety of approaches where music therapists theorise, describe, and propose diverse approaches, including trauma-informed approaches (Beck et al., 2018; Mallon and Antink, 2021; Parker et al., 2021), community approaches (Enge, 2015; Enge and Stige, 2022), culture-specific approaches (Abdulbaki and Berger, 2020), music psychotherapy approaches (Alanne, 2010), and music-centred approaches (Pavlicevic, 2003). In this chapter, our practice-led exploration of music therapy with children in transit camps focuses on a community-based psychosocial support approach which seems to best attend to the needs at hand. The time the children spend in a camp, where they reside temporarily, calls for music therapy to serve as a facilitating environment conducive to support, security, connection, and sharing.

The five years of music therapy groups in transit camps offered time and space for developing a unique perspective on the processes and actions required. This experience allowed for a combination of theoretical perspectives that would best address the physical, psychological, developmental, and social needs of refugee children. In particular, Mitsi's approach to group music therapy within the transit camps was (a) guided by the PFA principles, while informed by (b) an understanding of the neurobiological effect of trauma (van der Kolk, 2014), (c) an acceptance of the psychological strain of the refugee experience (Papadopoulos, 2019), and (d) an awareness of the impact of the environment on child development (Bronfenbrenner, 1979). This four-layered thinking focuses on various aspects of the psychosocial needs of the children.

Each person perceives, processes, and responds to external situations uniquely and individually, and the refugee experience does not, of course, have the same psychological impact on all (Papadopoulos, 2007). Being sensitive to the refugee experience by providing psychosocial support through music therapy—especially in the flight phase during which refugees are typically living in transit camps—boosts resilience, fosters security, enhances psychological strength, and focuses on positive qualities. According to the PFA principles, feelings of safety, calmness, connectedness, self and community efficacy, and hope are the main concerns of the music therapy sessions. By changing social conditions to create a space for people to feel safe, the provided environment allows them to thrive. In other words, an environment that fosters feelings of safety and trust is critical to calming the neural activity, which promotes self-regulation, and in turn fosters a healing process neurologically and beyond (van der Kolk, 2014). The music activities offered by Mitsi were informed by the neurobiology of trauma, and rhythm activities aimed at enhancing self-regulation. Self-regulation also develops through co-regulation, where empathetic and responsive interactions between the music therapist and the young participants fostered a supportive environment for expression of thoughts and understanding of emotions. The adversities presented in a transit refugee camp might have a strong impact on children's development, and group music therapy can prove beneficial in supporting a healthier sense of self.

Journey phase 4

During 2017, the number of unaccompanied refugee minors increased. In an effort to ensure their safety, a shelter away from the camps began to operate under the care of the NGO METADrasi. Towards the end of 2016, around 20 unaccompanied minors resided in that shelter. Mitsi provided weekly music therapy sessions for those living there and who expressed an interest to participate, for a duration of six months. The following vignette describes the fifth session that took place in the living room of the shelter.

Vignette 6 (Shelter for unaccompanied minors, October 25, 2016, Mitsi's fieldnotes)

A group of seven unaccompanied minors, three girls and four boys 11 to 14 years old, attended the music therapy group today. Some continue to have difficulty with keeping a steady rhythm, yet they all are beginning to sing louder and steadier. They enjoy improvising, sharing, and changing instruments, and they participate with group coordination and cohesion of sound in mind. They offer space, time, and support to each other, and, despite their cultural and ethnic differences, the environment created during the group is that of inclusivity.

On the one hand, the youngest in the group is an 11-year-old girl from Syria who seems to enjoy the session. She laughs often yet at the same time she is hesitant to use her singing voice. On the other hand, a 14-year-old boy from Syria, who does not seem to get along with the other children in the shelter; he participates while keeping some distance from the rest of the group. When the activities focused on emotions, the melodic instruments were used by all children to give voice to 'sadness' and the drums were used for 'anger' and/or 'joy.' Another 14-year-old boy from Syria stated that 'the glockenspiel is good for self-expression' and a 13-year-old girl from Kurdistan added: 'I can express myself better with the toubeleki and the glockenspiel.'

In addition to the shelter, a large number of unaccompanied refugee minors resided in the 'safe zone' in VIAL, yet without any psychosocial support. From 2017 to 2018, IOM funded a music therapy research project led by Mitsi for unaccompanied teenagers living on a temporary basis in VIAL's safe zone. The project lasted for about six months during which music therapy groups were provided weekly. A group of 12 teenagers participated, aged from 14 to 17, from 8 different countries (Afghanistan, Algeria, Eritrea, Guinea, Iraq, Kuwait, Palestine, and Syria), along with a cultural mediator/interpreter, a clinical psychologist, and a music therapist (Mitsi). The interventions used with this group were clinical improvisations, therapeutic drumming, singing, and songwriting. The following anonymised excerpt is from a focus group discussion facilitated by Mitsi following the last session. Attempting to give voice to the participants, these excerpts highlight their own perceptions of the music therapy groups.

Focus group (unedited and verbatim transcription, April 2, 2018)

Respondent 1: [In the music therapy groups] you know the others, the new people, the new friends.
Respondent 2: There I can express myself; you know, music is like... when you know music, you can say what you are feeling... it is very important, very important.
Mitsi: And you say you have this opportunity in this group to express yourself?
Respondent 2: Yes
Respondent 3: We were like one family, together, we had to cooperate together, and it was very nice for me.
Respondent 4: The music it does not mind if one is from Algeria, the other one from another country, all of us we were one country, we were together and its open mind at the same time
Respondent 5: Just, I have the same idea with what other people said, we are understanding, we are knowing new instruments, how to find sounds and new songs.
Mitsi: Do you want to share a difficulty you experienced?
Respondent 3: It was all very nice but still we don't know your name... Mitsi... Mitsi... [laughter]
Respondent 2: When we get confused, when we say our names, it is very funny for me, and I will never forget that.
Respondent 4: It was when we came, it was raining and the police stopped us and the police say that we cannot come, I will never forget that, I felt that... black... racist... and I will never forget that... I think this was because we are black... I will never forget that day... the police...

Even though all entry permits to the camps were secured well in advance, new police officers were never informed about the music therapy group, and we had to deal with authority issues most of the time, such as refusal of entrance, not allowing group members to join, or even asking to keep 'the noise level' low. In a hostile environment such as the safe zone, police can take on a quite threatening face in the eyes of refugees, and even more so for unaccompanied teenage refugees. In a group characterised by multiculturality, multiethnicity, and diversity in language and religion, music became an avenue where members could co-exist, co-operate, and share mutual musicking experiences. Music in this case fostered an environment for all to be together, sharing time, space, and sound.

Reflections, introspections, ways forward

The time of a person as a refugee in Chios can be described as being in limbo; waiting without a time chart. Life 'in limbo' (Ukrayinchuk and Havrylchyk, 2020, p. 1525) describes a long wait for asylum seeking papers to get processed, a time when refugees experience their present situation as characterised by a still movement and their lives on a temporary halt. During this time, refugee children are often neglected, hidden in the shadows of uncertainty and insecurity, and, as a result, are deprived of a healthy childhood. Without psychosocial, emotional, and educational support, children residing in transit camps come up against various adversities. The music therapy groups narrated above, reflect some aspects of the multifaceted reality faced in Chios since 2015 when the big refugee wave reached Europe. What we set out to do was to provide community music therapy as psychosocial support for refugee children, on a voluntary basis yet with professional diligence, consistency, and accountability.

The narratives presented earlier triggered self-reflection, questioning, and reassessment of the groups, the contexts, and the music therapy practices. Mitsi questioned, 'We volunteered and engaged empathetically, but did we actually help, since the adversities will not stop as refugees are here on a temporary basis, is providing a safe space for an hour or two enough? To what extent do we actually cover the psychosocial needs of refugee children?' (Mitsi's fieldnotes, 2020).

Providing group music therapy in transit camps that are in such a state of flux, presents various difficulties and uncertainties.

Vignette 7 (November 16, 2015, Mitsi's fieldnotes)

We did not go for a group today due to the funeral of young Ahmed who drowned coming to the island on Friday, November 11. Instead, we decided to attend the funeral. We are facing the sombre reality of difficult, unpredictable, and uncontrollable issues and we need to show the flexibility required to address them. It is important to be in tune with our pain as well, and the impact that the loss of children we will never meet has on us.

As written in the fieldnotes, that day we cancelled the group as there was the funeral of a refugee child who drowned at a boat accident five days ago. The communal grief of parents and siblings and the whole community of refugees affected our team of volunteers deeply. This and other similar experiences throughout our work highlighted the need to meet bi-weekly to reflect and support each other as a peer support group. This included our ways of coping with the lack of opportunities for predictable endings, since the departures of refugees from Chios were not planned well in advance. So, each group session had to provide some kind of closure for all participants, with wishes for a safe journey to those we would not perhaps see again.

From Mitsi's experience of providing community music therapy in transit camps, certain indications emerge that might be of value to other music therapists. Each person's need to feel safe and to trust the music therapy group should be acknowledged from the beginning. As Comte (2016) stresses, oftentimes we assume that refugee groups are homogeneous, yet safeguarding for each individual's needs is of paramount importance in transit settings, a period when the healthy development of children can be fragile and at risk. The use of the PFA principles can provide a larger framework for music therapy interventions as psychosocial support to this end.

Both knowing the context very well and being aware of the wider refugee experience are key to a music therapist's practice. Not all young people require specialist healthcare, and although literature tends to focus on refugees who are experiencing mental health needs, it seems important to pay attention to the person's everyday experience within a transit environment.

It is worth also considering the qualifications and training needed for music therapists serving as first aid responders in such contexts. In addition to a foundational music therapy training, it is vital for the practitioner to have some experience of community-oriented music therapy practices as well as PFA training. This includes an ability to meet individual needs within groups, an all-inclusive perspective, a critical reflexivity towards one's own limitations and biases, as well as a cultural and religious sensitivity and a sincere humanitarian interest. In addition, adopting a person-centred approach (McCormack and McCance, 2017) ensures that each individual is viewed holistically as a person, taking into account ethnic, religious, and cultural aspects of living.

In this chapter, we aimed to focus on the role of music therapy beyond a trauma limited focus and more in relation to the everyday refugee experience within transit camps where refugees live in a state of limbo. Community music therapy could be characterised as a low-intensity approach, adapting every time to the different contexts and individual needs of children (e.g., unaccompanied minors or children travelling with their parents, living in informal or organised camps with no educational or psychosocial activities, living confined within the hotspot) and striving to provide safety, opportunities for engagement as well as psychosocial and emotional support. Even though additional practice-led development and research in transit camps is needed, we propose that such an approach to music therapy has the potential to function on a proactive level ensuring a healthier environment for children within and in relation to their communities, as well as to boost resilience and promote their overall wellbeing.

Acknowledgements

We would like to express our sincere gratitude to Vicky Georgouli and Vassilis Pahoundakis for their permission to use the photographs included in the text as well as to the group of volunteers who participated and kept diaries during these years: Sevie Paida (educator), Despoina Armenaki (educator), Maria Kassapidou (arts teacher), and Kostas Sarrikostas (music teacher).

Notes

1 The autoharp (or autochord) is a strummed or plucked instrument. Its construction resembles a zither and chords are formed through the use of buttons which damp the strings not belonging to a chord each time.
2 Hotspots are first reception facilities promoted as a European strategy to manage migratory pressures in Greece and Italy.

References

Abdulbaki, H., and Berger, J. (2020). Using culture-specific music therapy to manage the therapy deficit of post-traumatic stress disorder and associated mental health conditions in Syrian refugee host environments. *Approaches: An Interdisciplinary Journal of Music Therapy*, 12(2): 211–223.

Akoyunoglou, M. (2019). The "Circle of Music" with refugee children in Chios Island: Description and reports of three years of field work. In T. Raptis and D. Koniari (Eds), *Music education and society: New challenges, new directions. Proceedings, 8th Conference of the Greek Society for Music Education*. Thessaloniki: GSME, pp. 94–101.

Alanne, S. (2010). Music psychotherapy with refugee survivors of torture. Interpretations of three clinical case studies. Sibelius Academy, Studia Musica 44. Music Education Department. Doctoral dissertation.

Beck, B. D., Lund, S. T., Søgaard, U., Simonsen, E., Tellier, T. C., Cordtz, T. O., Laier, G. H., and Moe, T. (2018). Music therapy versus treatment as usual for refugees diagnosed with posttraumatic stress disorder (PTSD): Study protocol for a randomized controlled trial. *Trials*, 19(1). doi:10.1186/s13063-018-2662-z.

Bensimon, M., Amir, D., and Wolf, Y. (2008). Drumming through trauma: Music therapy with post-traumatic soldiers. *The Arts in Psychotherapy*, 35(1): 34–48. doi:10.1016/j.aip.2007.09.002.

Betancourt, T. S., Frounfelker, R. L., Berent, J. M., Gautam, B., Abdi, S. M., Abdi, A. I., Haji, Z., Maalim, A., and Mishra, T. (2019). Addressing mental health disparities in refugee children through family and community-based prevention. In M. M. Suárez-Orozco (Ed), *Humanitarianism and mass migration: Confronting the world crisis*. Oakland, CA: California Scholarship Online, pp. 137–164.

Bronfenbrenner, U. (1979). *The ecology of human development: Experiments by nature and design*. Cambridge, MA, and London: Harvard University Press.

Cheng, K., and Zarinnegar, P. (2020). Children and adolescents. In J. D. Kinzie and G. A. Keepers (Eds), *The psychiatric evaluation and treatment of refugees*. Washington, DC: American Psychiatric Association Publishing, pp. 85–102.

Choi, C. M. H. (2010). A pilot analysis of the psychological themes found during the CARING at Columbia--music therapy program with refugee adolescents from North Korea. *Journal of Music Therapy*, 47(4): 380–407. doi:10.1093/jmt/47.4.380.

Comte, R. (2016). Neo-colonialism in music therapy: A critical interpretive synthesis of the literature concerning music therapy practice with refugees. *Voices: A World Forum for Music Therapy*, 16(3). 10.15845/voices.v16i3.865.

Council of the EU PRESS (2016). *EU-Turkey statement, 18 March 2016*. Press release. [online] Available at: https://www.consilium.europa.eu/en/press/press-releases/2016/03/18/eu-turkey-statement/pdf.

Crisp, J. (2009). Refugees, persons of concern, and people on the move: The broadening boundaries of UNHCR. *Refuge: Canada's Journal on Refugees*, [online] 26(1): 73–76. https://www.jstor.org/stable/48648349.

Daud, A., af Klinteberg, B., and Rydelius, P. A. (2008). Resilience and vulnerability among refugee children of traumatized and non-traumatized parents. *Child and Adolescent Psychiatry and Mental Health*, 2(7): 1–11. doi: 10.1186/1753-2000-2-7

Davis, K. M. (2010). Music and the expressive arts with children experiencing trauma. *Journal of Creative Mental Health*, 5: 125–133. doi: 10.1080/15401383.2010.485078

Dieltjens, T., Moonens, I., Van Praet, K., De Buck, E., and Vandekerckhove, P. (2014). A systematic literature search on psychological first aid: Lack of evidence to develop guidelines. *PLoS One*, 9(12): e114714. doi: 10.1371/journal.pone.0114714

Enge, K. E. A. (2015). Community music therapy with asylum-seeking and refugee children in Norway. *Journal of Applied Arts & Health*, 6(2): 205–215. doi: 10.13 86/jaah.6.2.205_1

Enge, K. E. A., & Stige, B. (2022). Musical pathways to the peer community: A collective case study of refugee children's use of music therapy. *Nordic journal of music therapy*, 31 (1), 7–24. doi: 10.1080/08098131.2021.1891130

Fox, M. (2002). Finding a way through: From mindlessness to minding. In R. Papadopoulos (Ed), *Therapeutic care for refugees: There is no place like home*. London: Karnac, pp. 103–120.

Garrido, S., Baker, F. A., Davidson, J. W., Moore, G., and Wasserman, S. (2015). Music and trauma: The relationship between music, personality, and comping style. *Frontiers in Psychology*, 6: 977. doi: 10.3389/fpsyg.2015.00977

Global Detention Project (2019). *Immigration detention in Greece: Stranded in Aegean limbo*. Country Report, September 2019. https://www.globaldetentionproject.org/greece-stranded-in-aegean-limbo

Gonzalez, M., Akoyunoglou, M., Sokira, J., Brooks, D., and Salgado, A. (2020). Music and music therapy in crises support interventions: Developing a global network. *Proceedings of the 16th WFMT World Congress of Music Therapy*, July 7–8, 2020, South Africa.

Heiderscheit, A., and Murphy, K. (2021). Trauma-informed care in music therapy: Principles, guidelines, and a clinical case illustration. *Music Therapy Perspectives*, 39(2): 142–151. doi: 10.1093/mtp/miab011

Hodes, M. (2019). New developments in the mental health of refugee children and adolescents. *Evidence-Based Mental Health*, 22: 72–76. doi: 10.1136/ebmental-2018-300065

Hodes, M., and Vostanis, P. (2019). Practitioner review: Mental health problems of refugee children and adolescents and their management. *The Journal of Child Psychology and Psychiatry*, 60(7): 716–731. doi: 10.1111/jcpp.13002

Kuriansky, J. (2019). A model psychosocial support training and workshop during a medical mission for Syrian refugee children in Jordan: Techniques, lessons learned and recommendations. *Journal of Infant, Child, and Adolescent Psychotherapy*, 18(4): 352–366. doi: 10.1080/15289168.2019.1690925

Mallon, T., and Hoog Antink, M. (2021). The sound of lost homes – Introducing the COVER model – Theoretical framework and practical insight into music therapy with refugees and asylum seekers. *Voices: A World Forum for Music Therapy*, 21(2). doi: 10.15845/voices.v21i2.3124

Map of Chios Island, Greece (2022). Image from Google Maps, accessed May 20, 2022. https://www.google.com/maps/@38.4194506,26.3950486,10z

McCormack, B., and McCance, T. (2017). *Person-centred practice in nursing and health care: Theory and practice*. 2nd ed. Chichester: Wiley Blackwell.

McFerran, K., and Teggelove, K. (2011). Music therapy with young people in schools: After the Black Saturday fires. *Voices: A World Forum for Music Therapy*, 11(1). doi: 10.15845/voices.v11i1.285

Motti-Stefanidi, F., Pavlopoulos, V., Papathanasiou, N., and Mastrotheodoros, S. (2020). Resilient adaptation of migrant and teenage refugees: Who is doing well and why? *Psychology: Journal of the Greek Psychological Association*, 25(1): 20–34. doi: 10.12681/psy_hps.25334

Papadopoulos, R. (2002). Refugees, home and trauma. In R. Papadopoulos (Ed), *Therapeutic care for refugees: There is no place like home*. London: Karnac, pp. 9–39.

Papadopoulos, R. (2007). Refugees, trauma and adversity – Activated development. *European Journal of Psychotherapy and Counselling*, 9(3): 301–312. doi: 10.1080/13642530701496930

Papadopoulos, R. (2018). An uncertain safety: Integrative health care for the 21st century refugees. *European Journal of Psychotraumatology*, 9(1). doi: 10.1080/20008198.2018.1549

Papadopoulos, R. (Ed) (2019). *Psychosocial dimensions of the refugee condition. The Synergic Approach* [in Greek]. Athens: Babel Centre for Refugees and Centre for Trauma, Asylum and Refugees.

Papadopoulos, R. (2021). *Involuntary dislocation: Home, trauma, resilience, and adversity-activated development*. New York, NY: Routledge.

Parker, D., Younes, L., Orabi, M., Procter, S., and Paulini, M. (2021). Music therapy as a protection strategy against toxic stress for Palestinian refugee children in Lebanon: A pilot research study. *Approaches: An Interdisciplinary Journal of Music Therapy*, 1–23.

Pavlicevic, M. (2003). *Groups in music: Strategies from music therapy*. London: Jessica Kingsley Publishers.

Poulos, C. N. (2021). Conceptual foundations of autoethnography. In C. N. Poulos (Ed), *Essentials of autoethnography*. Washington, DC: American Psychological Association, pp. 3–17. doi: 10.1037/0000222-001

Reyes, A. (1999). *Songs of the caged, songs of the free: Music and the Vietnamese refugee experience*. Philadelphia, PA: Temple University Press.

Shultz, J. M., and Forbes, D. (2013). Psychological first aid: Rapid proliferation and the search for evidence. *Disaster Health*, 2(1): 3–12. doi: 10.4161/dish.26006

Storsve, V., Westbye, I. A., and Ruud, E. (2010). Hope and recognition: A music project among youth in a Palestinian refugee camp. *Voices: A World Forum for Music Therapy*, 10(1). doi: 10.15845/voices.v10i1.158

Sutton, J. (Ed) (2002). *Music, music therapy and trauma: International perspectives*. London: Jessica Kingsley Publishers.

van der Kolk, B. (2014). *The body keeps the score: Brain, mind and body in the healing of trauma*. New York, NY: Penguin Random House LLC.

Ukrayinchuk, N., and Havrylchyk, O. (2020). Living in limbo: Economic and social costs for refugees. *Canadian Journal of Economics/Revue canadienne d' économique*, 53: 1523–1551. doi: 10.1111/caje.12475

UNHCR (2017). *Greece data snapshot: 13 March 2017*. United Nations High Commissioner for Refugees. https://data2.unhcr.org/en/documents/download/54451

Vaghri, Z., Tessier, Z., and Whalen, C. (2019). Refugee and asylum-seeking children: Interrupted child development and unfulfilled child rights. *Children*, 6(11): 120. doi: 10.3390/children6110120

Wang, L., Norman, I., Xiao, T., Li, Y., and Leamy, M. (2021). Psychological first aid training: A scoping review of its application, outcomes and implementation. *International Journal of Environmental Research and Public Health*, 18: 4594. doi: 10.3390/ijerph18094594

Weissbecker, I., Hanna, F., El Shazly, M., Gao, J., and Ventevogel, P. (2019). Integrative mental health and psychosocial support interventions for refugees in humanitarian crisis settings. In T. Wezel & B. Droždek (Eds), *An uncertain safety: Integrative health care for the 21st century refugees*. Cham: Springer, pp. 117–154.

Yayan, E. H., Düken, M. E., Özdemir, A. A., and Çelebioğlu, A. (2020). Mental health problems of Syrian refugee children: Post-traumatic stress, depression and anxiety. *Journal of Pediatric Nursing*, 51: e27–e32. doi: 10.1016/j.pedn.2019.06.012

Chapter 3

Music therapy and dramatherapy in children's hospices

'Playing in time'

Sarah Hodkinson and Gloria Garbujo

Introduction

Palliative care for children and young people is currently defined as 'an active and total approach to care, embracing physical, emotional, social and spiritual elements. It focuses on enhancement of quality of life for the child and support for the family and includes the management of distressing symptoms, provision of respite, and care following death and in bereavement' (Hain et al., 2021: 28). As for the individual needs of young people with life-limiting conditions, the definition of paediatric palliative care is evolving with time. Conceptual boundaries are constantly challenged by the changing needs of young people, requiring the reconfiguration of meanings within the therapeutic relationship and the creation of new ways of working beyond the traditional therapeutic space.

In this chapter, the authors reflect on their experience of facilitating music therapy and dramatherapy interventions at Shooting Star Children's Hospices (SSCH) (Shooting Star Children's Hospices, 2023). The two vignettes demonstrate how 'playing in time' with the needs of young people required the therapists to continually revisit the boundaries of clinical practice. Through a phenomenological approach, the authors explore the specific needs of adolescents and their desire to share their story. Themes of identity, intersubjectivity, and legacy are pivotal, with the creative material supporting a narrative process within the therapeutic interventions (Romanoff and Thompson, 2006).

The cultural context for this investigation is the United Kingdom, where the hospice movement started in 1967, and the first children's hospice opened in 1982 (Armstrong-Dailey and Zarbock, 2008). Paediatric palliative care remains a relatively new area of care, constantly evolving and adapting to medical and cultural changes. In the UK, arts therapies (art therapy, music therapy, and dramatherapy) are widely practised in children's hospices as a form of psychological therapy (Hodkinson et al., 2014). Arts therapists are qualified mental health professionals registered with the Health and Care Professions Council (HCPC, 2023).

DOI: 10.4324/9781003265610-4

Children's hospices provide holistic care for children and young people with life-limiting conditions and their families from the moment of diagnosis, throughout the trajectory of the illness, during end of life, and typically with three years of bereavement care. Life-limiting conditions are those for which there is no reasonable hope of cure and where premature death is inevitable. Some of these conditions cause progressive deterioration, often resulting in children and young people becoming increasingly dependent on their parents and carers (Together for Short Lives, 2022). The services provided at SSCH follow the ICPN (International Children's Palliative Care Network) charter (ICPN, 2022), which sets the standards of support for young people living with life-limiting conditions. The charter identifies education, play, and culturally appropriate psychosocial support as key to relieving existential distress. There is an emphasis on addressing the specific needs of young people in their transition to adulthood, encouraging participation in decision-making according to their age and understanding.

Setting

SSCH is made up of four clinical services: a hospice bedded unit, a community nursing team, a specialist symptom care team, and a multi-professional family support service. These four services offer support to approximately 700 families through cross-team, multi-disciplinary forums where family need and provision are considered carefully. Young people in SSCH's care may be at a deteriorating or end of life phase of illness and require specialist care from all four services to meet their physical, emotional, and social needs. Young people may outlive their life-limiting prognosis and move into adulthood, requiring services such as adult health, social care, education, employment, and housing. UK authorities begin supporting the transition of young people with additional needs when they are 14 years old (NICE, 2016). SSCH offers a transition case worker to each young person, to help navigate the practical and psychological complexities that exist when a young person and family transition from children's hospice care. Often young people experience periods of stable health, in which they may draw on SSCH's psychological support to manage day-to-day challenges.

Music therapy, dramatherapy, and art therapy are provided by the therapists of the Family Support Service. These can also be accessed by family members (siblings, guardians, and grandparents). Following the initial referral, the assessment phase is arranged with the young person and their parents. This is a collaborative process aimed at determining whether therapy is timely and appropriate, clarifying what problems could be addressed during the intervention. Where appropriate, a series of sessions is arranged with regular reviews of outcomes. Feedback forms and standardised questionnaires are used to evaluate and monitor progress. Alongside individual, dyadic, and family therapy, the therapists facilitate support groups, such as therapeutic workshops containing music and storytelling activities exploring themes of loss and resilience, providing opportunities for shared personal experience and learning coping strategies (Chin et al., 2018).

The diagnosis of a life-limiting condition produces 'a dividing line, a marker of "before and after" and ruptures the continuity between the past, present, and future' (Sourkes, 2007: 38). It is coupled with an unwelcome companion known as anticipatory grief, which is sorrow that is felt as losses are anticipated before the actual death. Families adjust to several changes in their daily routine and cope with symbolic and material loss during the illness trajectory. In times of crisis, young people can become acutely aware of the emotional distress experienced by their parents and their siblings. Adults are often perceived as role models, and their communication patterns can determine how well young people cope with their condition (Brown and Warr, 2003).

Young people's perception of death varies depending on cognitive development, the degree to which daily activities can be performed, the progression and severity of the symptoms, and communication within the family. Depending on the phase of the illness and how the body is affected, death anxiety can be acutely present in young people and difficult to address. Where families experience difficulties in communication about death and dying, there are higher risks of young people developing dysfunctional coping strategies, behavioural difficulties, and self-harming behaviours (Carter, 2016). On the contrary, talking through worries and fears about death can help young people feel less isolated and create opportunities to assign meaning to the experiences of loss caused by the illness (Stein et al., 2019).

Therapeutic interventions utilising the arts can help young people living with life-limiting conditions to express and manage their emotions, process traumatic experiences, and enhance a sense of legacy (Boucher et al., 2014). Depending on young people's needs and cognitive abilities, difficulties can be addressed verbally or explored non-verbally and indirectly using metaphor and imagery. During legacy-making activities, young people can create artworks representing aspects of themselves and ask their loved ones to treasure their creations. Sharing autobiographical songs and stories through legacy-making facilitates the process of coming to terms with loss (O'Callaghan, 2013). Recent studies on anticipatory grief and bereavement show that the use of metaphor helpfully allows individuals to 're-establish a coherent self-narrative that integrates the loss, while also permitting their life story to move forward along new lines' (Neimeyer et al., 2010: 78). Therapists at SSCH work alongside families helping them to integrate feelings of loss through legacy-making activities, providing parenting advice, supporting communication about death and dying and suggesting creative strategies for emotional regulation.

During the past five years, there has been a surge in referrals describing existing mental health difficulties, a surge that is reflected worldwide (Kieling et al., 2011). At the onset of COVID-19, statutory mental health services were stretched further, and access difficulties for young people reached a crisis. The urgency and anxiety about accessing support are felt strongly, as these mental health treatments offered by charitable services, such as SSCH, have become a lifeline to young people in palliative care. The following clinical vignettes demonstrate how two therapists navigated these challenges, 'playing in time' with the needs of young people. The first vignette presents a hospice-based music therapy intervention in which therapeutic songwriting is utilised to share a sense of self. The second vignette describes a dramatherapy intervention rich in self-discovery through storymaking. This was facilitated mostly online by virtual means, necessitated by the COVID-19 pandemic in which the hospice adapted to the needs of the population at the time. A full examination of the potential and limitations of online arts therapies is beyond the purpose of this article, but further exploration can be found in relevant articles (Feniger-Schaal et al., 2022).

Vignette 1: Amyas' songwriting process in music therapy

Amyas was referred to SSCH when he was eight years old and, against expectation, graduated from children's hospice care aged 21 years old. Amyas is a young person that staff and families had a great fondness for, enjoying sharing in his excitement about life and getting to know his thoughtful and charismatic personality. When he was 16 years old, a hospice nurse asked Amyas' parents if he needed support coping with his illness and disability and the impact on his mental health, to which a referral for therapy was actioned, and therapy commenced. A second 12-month intervention took place when he was 18 due to lowered mood and increased behavioural episodes.

Amyas lives with Lesch-Nyhan syndrome (LNS), a rare genetic condition caused by the absence, or near-absence, of the enzyme *hypoxanthine-guanine phosphoribosyltransferase* (Nguyen and William, 2016). Depending on the phenotype of this condition, a varying picture of neurological and behavioural abnormalities exists. The most striking of these for Amyas were involuntary movements and self-injurious behaviours such as hitting his head with his fist, biting his hand, and placing his fingers in his throat to cause gagging and bleeding. Self-mutilation is very much the hallmark symptom of LNS (Deon et al., 2011), though not true for Amyas. Self-injurious behaviours and self-mutilation can bring significant emotional challenge to the individual and to caregivers watching an internal struggle take place as a loved one tries to fight against this powerful compulsion. Amyas had a deep brain stimulator in situ to lessen behavioural symptoms, and he chose to have his hands in mittens, kept strapped to the side of his wheelchair to lessen incidents in which others were hurt by his involuntary movements. In his therapy, it became evident that LNS also induces emotional self-injurious behaviours such as the destruction of attachments and mistruths that would lead to anger towards him from loved ones and carers. The condition is relentless and unforgiving.

Amyas had a great passion for music and in particular singing, leading to an immediate desire to engage with music-making in his sessions. From the moment sessions began, the relationship represented that of co-musicians enjoying the art form together through discussing artists, instruments, and Amyas' musical ambitions. In parallel to this, the therapist was given insight into his world, learning about what it felt like to live with LNS, his life-limiting condition. Amyas revealed a joyful character, determined to be known, to be famous, and to be heard, along with the unenviable psychological struggles of adolescence, further complicated by a deeply debilitating disability. His parents told the therapist that despite a joyful exterior, there was an inner unhappiness and struggle. In a hospice movement that so passionately wishes to disregard the disability and make everyday family-life experiences possible, without psychological therapies, there is a danger that the pain and inner turmoil can be left without a voice. Amyas used the therapeutic space to give this a voice.

Amyas' narrative became one of heroes and heroines. These took the shape of his girlfriend (a class-mate), his teaching assistant, hospice staff (usually the younger females), and various famous characters and music artists such as James Bond and John Legend. Amyas had deep affection for others. His excitement to see or talk about one of his heroes often led to emotional dysregulation that caused an immediate exacerbation of distressing involuntary movements and self-injurious behaviours. Amyas' ambition was to feature in Simon Cowell's television production 'The X-Factor,' but even discussing this triggered an attack. The therapist and Amyas created a behavioural strategy to help Amyas identify his arousal level beginning to increase. When Amyas felt this change of state, he used 'amber' to describe a move away from his calm state 'green' before a physiological and uncontrollable 'red' reaction ensued. This allowed the therapist to support Amyas in self-regulating with significant success. However, this emotional rollercoaster of elation and frustration was exhausting for Amyas, and as Valentine's Day approached, Amyas' desire for his voice to be heard grew. To contain this, the therapist suggested Amyas compose his first song, which he dedicated to his girlfriend and titled 'Love.'

'Love' (verse 1)
She comes, into the room
I can't help but smile at her
She's looking, up to me
For love, for love
She's beautiful, she's beautiful
She's beautiful, she's beautiful

The following week, Amyas asked for a video recording of the song to be taken to his girlfriend who was staying at the hospice. After a quick assessment of risk, this took place, and his girlfriend, who is profoundly disabled and unable to communicate verbally, responded instantaneously with a beaming smile and turned her gaze to Amyas. The moment shared by several hospice staff felt incredibly special. Amyas' artistry grew, and his desire to share his song grew more and more, requiring the therapist to give careful thought to emotional vulnerability, safety, and the desires of young people.

When confidence plummets in adolescence, individual identity is often built on talents, interests, and fascinations. For Amyas, therapeutic songwriting became his expertise and a vehicle for expression. A pad of manuscript became the source of ideas for topics, titles, and lyrics. Then positioned at the centre of the room with a microphone in place, Amyas choreographed each song, choosing between acoustic and electric guitars, selecting a favourite from chord patterns offered, melodic line suggestions, and possible organisation of lyrics. Though at first, the therapist supported with example frameworks, over time Amyas' choices grew in speed and confidence. Depending on how he presented at the start of each session, the therapist could determine what level of support was required from the songwriting partnership. When low in mood, this was acknowledged with care, delicately and slowly offering space and snippets of musical ideas. When elated, the songs became a needed emotional container. Themes of power, rage, adoration, and affection flooded the songs. Therapeutic song composition became a winning formula to hold and express Amyas' thematic material in a deep and profound way.

Living in world where the sharing of content is often immediate, Amyas passionately wished to share every recording at the end of every session with everyone! The therapist offered opportunities to help Amyas slowly and carefully manage opportunities for sharing his material, as well as opportunities to debrief together, exploring the psychological impact of doing so. This became a key strategy that also protected the therapeutic intervention creating a bubble of confidentiality for several weeks between performances, in order that themes could safely arise and be explored within the confidential therapeutic space. Most remarkable to the therapist was that Amyas' musical choices demonstrated a mature musicianship in which creative choices were repeatedly brilliant in their artistic property. Each pop song and ballad Amyas created was as catchy as the previous one, with a likeable quality and powerful meaning drawn from Amyas' unique life experience (Figure 3.1).

Amyas built a bank of songs over several months to create his first album of nine compositions and then went on to create a second album. A photoshoot was organised, and album-release events were created in the hospice in which pre-agreed samples were shared. Amyas gave careful thought to which staff to invite. He created songs and covers versions to perform at the

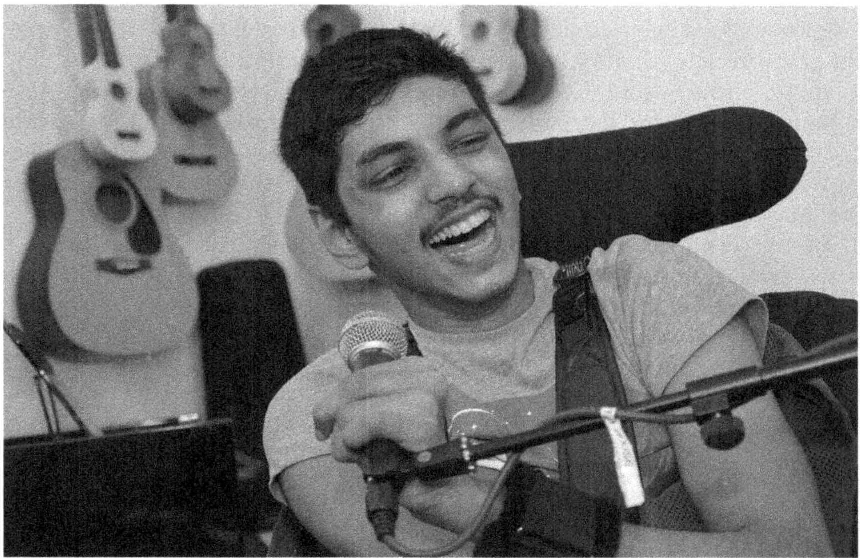

Figure 3.1 Photo of Amyas featuring on his album cover.

hospice Christmas carol concert to great acclaim. After spending time reflecting on his experience of sharing his song 'Love' in the privacy of the hospice, with parental consent, he was given the opportunity to meet with the hospice public relations and communications team to share the story on the SSCH website, social media platforms and in local media sources.

It comes as no surprise that the therapist was challenged by fierce protection of the client and the therapeutic space versus needing to 'play in time' with the fast-paced needs of young people, who are immersed in daily releases of self-made music videos, imagery, and content. This content has become a voice for young people in the world and a means to connect. Therapy invites a young person to find a voice and can sensitively and meaningfully help bring this voice into the world.

Vignette 2: Noor's storymaking process in online dramatherapy

This vignette describes a dramatherapy intervention with a young girl named Noor, who was 12 at the time of the sessions, and her mother, Faridah. The referral had been made by a paediatric nurse in the Community Team at SSCH. In the referral, Noor was described as a bright girl who was experiencing anxiety and low mood in relation to muscular dystrophy, a genetic condition characterised by progressive muscle weakness (Roland, 2000).

Following the referral, in agreement with Noor and Faridah, a dramatherapy assessment commenced. The process involved two parent meetings and three conjoint therapy sessions with Noor and Faridah. Due to the lockdown measures in COVID-19 and transport difficulties, these were conducted online. At the end of the therapy assessment, when it became apparent that further support was needed and that online sessions were suitable for Noor, weekly sessions continued online, with careful thought given to safety and effectiveness.

The intervention lasted 11 months, with some breaks during school time, and it involved one face-to-face session at the hospice towards the end of the process. At that stage, Noor was able to express her desire to share the dramatherapy process with others and make it 'visible' so that other young people could benefit from it. By 'playing in time' with Noor's evolving needs, the final part of the dramatherapy intervention focused on the creation of a piece of writing, which was then adapted for the edition of 'Shine' (SSCH's magazine) and shared on SSCH's social media account and website (Shooting Star Children's Hospices, 2022), as agreed with Noor and Faridah.

The account below is based on the original version created during the sessions with Noor. It describes the dramatherapy process and has been included in this book chapter with Noor and Faridah's consent. It is an example of the use of storymaking and projective techniques (Millbrook, 2019) to support young people in developing and sharing their own story in the way they wish (Figure 3.2).

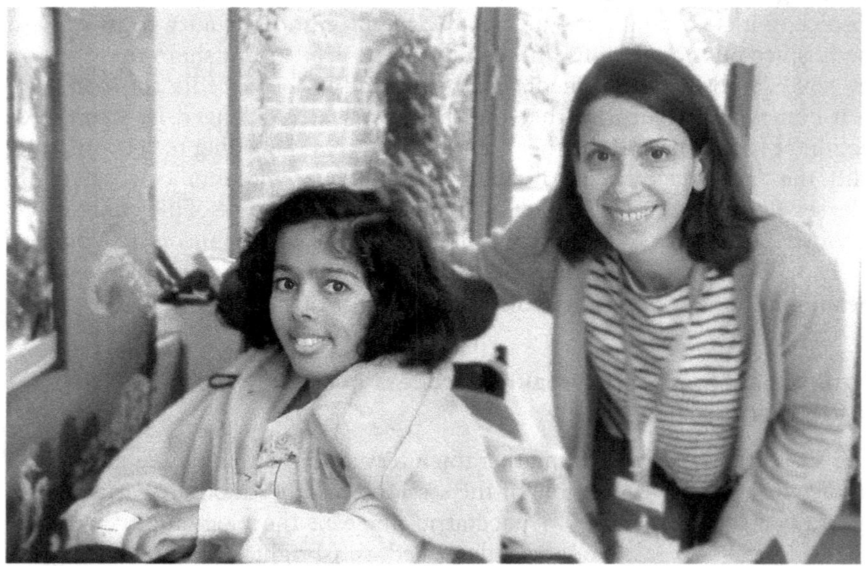

Figure 3.2 Photo of Noor and the dramatherapist at Shooting Star Children's Hospices.

Noor's dramatherapy sessions (via Zoom) started in March 2021, during the COVID-19 pandemic, with the aim of helping Noor express her emotions and increase her confidence. At that time arranging social activities presented as extremely challenging, and Noor was able to share with the therapist the sense of isolation and sadness that she was experiencing due to the limited number of interactions with her friends and her favourite teacher. In addition, the date for Noor's surgery was approaching and dramatherapy allowed Noor to express her fears and worries about the treatment. As Noor later described, the sessions helped her so that she was 'not feeling scared when the day of the surgery arrived.'

During her initial sessions, Noor and the therapist started to get to know each other through creative techniques and games. Noor's mother, Faridah, joined the appointments helping with art materials and practical activities. At that time, Noor's desire to create a story based on her own experiences became evident, and with the support of her therapist and her mother, she engaged in a storymaking process. Noor presented with exceptional artistic and storytelling skills, and the most natural way for her to start creating her story was through drawing. The structure of the drawing was inspired by a dramatherapy technique called 'Six-part story method (6PSM)' (Lahad et al., 2013), which is particularly useful for assessing resilience and coping strategies through symbolic expression.

Noor created 'Luna in the jungle,' a story about 'Luna,' a girl diagnosed with a complex genetic condition which prevented her from walking. Luna was a 'kind, caring, confident, and brave girl,' and throughout the story, she discovered her strengths and 'super-powers.' At the start of the story, Luna found herself lost in the jungle, but fortunately, her friends, the animals, protected her and helped her face different challenges. Eventually, Luna found her way back home and reunited with her parents. Noor's favourite part of the story was 'when Luna goes to the cave and finds the key to open the magic door,' a moment which represented Luna's process of self-discovery and self-empowerment. After completing the different parts of the drawing, Noor and the therapist decided to write down the story by sharing their screens on Zoom and looking at the document together. The writing process presented as extremely exciting for Noor and she started typing new paragraphs in between sessions.

During the summer holidays Noor and the therapist decided 'to bring the story to life,' and Noor, with the help of her mother Faridah, was able to create an exceptional puppet theatre using a shoe box, cutting out the characters, and sticking them to cardboard. As Noor described later, making the theatre and preparing for the puppet show was her favourite part of the whole storymaking process. When the puppet show was ready, Noor invited her younger brother to the session, asking him to help her move the puppets and 'be the puppeteers together.'

In the following weeks, Noor explained to the therapist her idea of transforming the story into a video game, with the help of her older brother who was passionate about coding. In between sessions, Noor asked her brother to teach her how to make the code for the story using a children's website called 'Tynker.' During the following sessions, Noor shared on Zoom the first chapter of the story ... transformed into a video game! Noor's mother described feelings of intense surprise in seeing all the different characters interacting and re-enacting the story online. In that moment Noor expressed her desire to show her creations, publicly, to other families at SSCH. As Noor said 'in this way other children can create their own stories,' based on their own experiences.

In the Autumn, Noor, Faridah, and the therapist met at the hospice for the first time. Noor's family lived far from the hospice, but the professionals were able to arrange transport for an in-person session. Noor brought her puppet theatre and re-told the story with the help of the therapist. Before the end of the session, they said goodbye and celebrated the process by improvising with musical instruments and taking some photos together. Noor described the appointment as 'a very special session.'

During the following sessions on Zoom, Noor and the therapist looked back at the therapeutic intervention, focusing on the creations that Noor had made. They also decided to write a brief account of the storymaking process to acknowledge the positive changes that happened during the months they worked together. As agreed with Noor and Faridah the piece of writing was then adapted for SSCH magazine and website, as well as social media platforms.

At the end of the intervention, Faridah acknowledged that Noor's confidence had increased significantly, and the process had helped Noor express her feelings through the art form. As Faridah has described: 'the sessions have been incredible because they helped Noor waking up her creativity ... Maybe Noor she did not know that she could write stories and create videogames ... but eventually she did! And she got a lot of ideas out of the sessions, so she can do more things!'.

Discussion

Adolescence is a period of deep transformation, turmoil, and change, a time of experimentation and self-discovery. When working with young people whose mental health suffers from the consequences of a medicalised life and the sense of uncertainty related to a life-limiting condition, it is essential to adopt a non-pathologising approach (Coleman and Kelly, 2017). From a phenomenological perspective, this approach provides space to consider young people's narratives about their conditions in relationship with the world in which they are situated, incorporating concepts such as gender, race, culture, sexuality, and spirituality.

The impact of a life-limiting illness on the development of body image, emotional independence, and sexual expression is difficult to measure fully.

There may be repeated hospital admissions and frequent episodes of pain. School absence and limited social interactions often have adverse consequences on self-esteem and confidence. Conditions which pose a limit in physical abilities or alter appearance are often experienced with a sense of frustration and failure during social interactions with their peers (Rodriguez et al., 2018). Social difficulties have a significant effect on emotional health and well-being.

The vignettes presented in this chapter show Amyas and Noor's desire to engage in legacy-making activities and maintain autonomy and vision over the creative process through songwriting and storymaking. Both Amyas and Noor have voiced their desire to share their creations, achieved within the therapeutic intervention, via social media and other contexts at SSCH. They wished for their stories and voices to be heard, validated, and shared within a caring community and beyond.

Sharing material from a session is a delicate matter requiring clinical supervision and great consideration of what the long-term emotional impact might be and the implications for a confidential therapeutic space. In particular, for a young person with a condition that affects cognition and development, the capacity to understand the impact must be assessed and until adulthood, the consent of parents is sought. Some young people with developmental disabilities, or presenting as neurodivergent, often compare their way of moving, thinking, and talking to what neurotypical growth should look like and also to the way of being and communicating of famous artists and their cult heroes. This can cause a profound sense of frustration and requires greater honesty, courage, and capacity to tolerate envy in order to find their own way to navigate adolescence and express their full potential (Sinason, 1992).

Alongside Amyas and Noor's desire to be seen was their greater longing to belong, and this was set against the painful reality of how remarkably different they felt compared to their peers. What emerged in therapy was that belonging today in a society that celebrates individuality, does not have to be about being the same as others. Belonging can be about finding your narrative and being heard. Amyas' powerful series of autobiographical songs and Noor's autobiographical puppet show captured their experiences and enabled them to belong to a digital age where personal stories, through social media and other online channels, become opportunities to champion values that are not often present in society.

Whether the immense significance or depth of Amyas and Noor's creations is ever fully understood outside of the therapeutic space, is a question that remains unanswered. Perhaps, this is equally true for every professional artist who draws deeply on personal experience. Similarly, whether the balance of holding a confidential space for their clients and sharing material publicly was exactly right throughout the therapeutic processes will always be a question that sits with the therapists. Perhaps, like parenting an adolescent, it represents the metaphorical dance between providing protection and enabling independence.

Conclusion

Within an individualistic culture where the ideology of mental illness has become dominant, recent studies have stressed how cost-based decisions have led to an alarming agenda in mental health care, essentially focused on productivity as a health outcome (Isham et al., 2020). In the context of paediatric palliative care, this is highlighted by the biomedicine hegemonic discourse, where caring for young people without being able to cure their conditions can be perceived as a process destined to fail. As a culture, we tend to address health and illness through a medicalised approach and consider death taboo; however, palliative care aims to embrace physical, spiritual, social, and emotional aspects within an integrative approach (Testoni et al., 2021).

The arts therapies provide an invaluable space to address pertinent themes of identity, intersubjectivity, and legacy in young people living with a life-limiting condition. A holding and facilitative environment can help young people build an authentic relationship with the therapist and express their emotions through the art form. Therapists can help young people identify their own strategies to cope with the transitions they face and support them in making informed choices in relation to their relationships, their future, and their care plan. This chapter has shown how creative techniques can be crucial when working with young people with cognitive and developmental issues.

Perhaps more deeply, as professionals it is essential to acknowledge how ability and disability can be considered as identity parameters (Dokter and Sajnani, 2023) and to help young people re-construct narratives concerning these concepts. During the COVID-19 pandemic and the restriction applied because of the global health emergency, personal stories of marginalisation have become significantly present in the therapeutic space. By adopting a phenomenological approach to this subject, it could be argued that:

> [...] the question about human body is bound to the question about human *finitude*. Finitude can be understood negatively, as the *limits of agency* rooted in the intrinsic restrictiveness of the body. [...] Alternatively, finitude can be understood positively, as the *contextual embeddedness* of human being, including human perceiving, thinking, feeling, and acting (Mladenov, 2016: 57).

From a therapeutic perspective, 'playing in time' with Amyas and Noor's needs has challenged the boundaries of clinical practice, expanding the creative process outside the therapeutic space. It is the authors' sense that when therapists revisit and challenge therapeutic boundaries, young people may be able to re-establish trust and encounter other parts of themselves. Young people may choose to become authors, directors, and performers and invite therapists to play the roles of witness, audience, and co-performer.

From a phenomenological perspective, the self-narratives presented in this chapter can be described as evolving creations within an intersubjective matrix (Pitruzzella, 2016). Through songwriting and storymaking, Noor and Amyas have become advocates for the needs of young people living with life-limited conditions and championed the themes of inclusion and diversity for other young people facing similar challenges.

Music therapy and dramatherapy in children's hospices, in their participatory and collaborative nature, can provide the opportunity to re-signify personal stories and encourage a change of narratives in society. Ultimately, to 'play in time' with the needs of young people living with a life-limiting condition constantly requires a look at the concept of identity in a more relational approach, allowing new meanings to emerge from the therapeutic relationship and to change over time.

References

Armstrong-Dailey, A., and Zarbock, S. (Eds) (2008). *Hospice care for children*. Oxford: Oxford University Press.

Boucher, S., Downing, J., and Shemilt, R. (2014). The role of play in children's palliative care. *Children*, 1(3), pp. 302–317.

Brown, E., and Warr, B. (2003). *Supporting the child and the family in paediatric palliative care*. London: Jessica Kingsley Publisher.

Carter, M. (2016). *Helping children and adolescents think about death, dying and bereavement*. London: Jessica Kingsley Publishers.

Chin, W. L., Jaaniste, T., and Trethewie, S. (2018). The role of resilience in the sibling experience of Pediatric Palliative Care: What is the theory and evidence? *Children*, 5(7), pp. 97–107.

Coleman, A., and Kelly, A. (2017). Two to one. In R. Hougham and B. Jones (Eds), *Dramatherapy: Reflections and praxis*. London: Routledge, pp. 123–143.

Deon, L. L., Kalichman, M. A., Booth, C. L., Slavin, K. V., and Deborah J., Gaebler-Spira (2011). Pallidal deep-brain stimulation associated with complete remission of self-injurious behaviors in a patient with Lesch-Nyhan syndrome: A case report. *Journal of Child Neurology*, 27(1), pp. 117–120.

Dokter, D., and Sajnani, S. (2023). *Intercultural dramatherapy. Imagination and action at the intersections of difference*. London: Routledge.

Feniger-Schaal, R., Orkibi, H., Keisari, S., Sajnani, N. L., and Butler, J. B. (2022). Shifting to tele-creative arts therapies during the COVID-19 pandemic: An international study on helpful and challenging factors. *The Arts in Psychotherapy*, 78, p. 101898.

Hain, R., Goldman, A., Rapoport, A., and Meiring, M. (Eds) (2021). *Oxford textbook of paediatric palliative care (3edn)*. Oxford: Oxford University Press.

Hodkinson, S., Bunt, L., and Daykin, N. (2014). Music therapy in children's hospices: An evaluative survey of provision. *The Arts in Psychotherapy*, 41, pp. 570–576.

International children's palliative care network (2022). *The ICPN charter*. Available at: https://www.icpcn.org/icpcn-charter/ (Accessed 18.12.2022)

Isham, A., Mair, S., and Jackson, T. (2020). *Wellbeing and productivity: A review of the literature*. Centre for the Understanding of Sustainable Prosperity. CUSP Working Paper Series. No 22. Guildford: University of Surrey.

Kieling, C., Baker-Henningham, H., Belfer, M., Conti, G., Ertem, I., Omigbodum, O., Rohde, L. A., Srinath, S., Ulkeur, N., and Rahman, A. (2011). Child and adolescent mental health worldwide: Evidence for action. *Lancet*, 378, pp. 1515–1525.

Lahad, M., Shacham, M., and Ayalon, O. (2013). The "Basic Ph" model of coping and resiliency. *Theory, research and cross-cultural applications*. London: Jessica Kingsley Publisher.

Millbrook, A. (2019). Digital storymaking: Dramatherapy with young people online. *Dramatherapy*, 40(1), pp. 28–40.

Mladenov, T. (2016). *Critical theory and disability. A phenomenological approach*. London: Bloomsbury.

National Institute for Health and Care Excellence (2016). *Transition from children's to adult's services for young people using health or social care services. NICE guideline* [NG43] Available at: https://www.nice.org.uk/guidance/ng43 (Accessed 23.03.2023)

Neimeyer, R. A., Burke, L. A., Mackay, M. M., and Van Dyke Stringer, J. G. (2010). Grief therapy and the reconstruction of meaning: From principles to practice. *Journal of Contemporary Psychotherapy*, 40, 73–83.

Nguyen, K. V., and William, L. N. (2016). Mutation in the human HPRT1 gene and the Lesch-Nyhan syndrome. *Nucleosides, Nucleotides and Nucleic Acids*, 35(8), pp. 426–434.

O'Callaghan, C. (2013). Music therapy preloss care though legacy creation. *Progress in Palliative Care*, 21(2), pp. 78–82.

Pitruzzella, S. (2016). *Drama, creativity and intersubjectivity: The roots of change in Dramatherapy*. London: Routledge.

Rodriguez, A., Smith, J., and McDermid, K. (2018). Dignity therapy interventions for young people in palliative care: A rapid structured evidence review. *International Journal of Palliative Nursing*, 24(7), pp. 339–349.

Roland, E. H. (2000). Muscular dystrophy. *Journal of Pediatrics Review*, 21(7), pp. 233–237.

Romanoff, B. D., and Thompson, B. E. (2006). Meaning construction in palliative care: The use of narrative, ritual, and the expressive arts. *American Journal of Hospice & Palliative Medicine*, 23(4), pp. 309–316.

Shooting Star Children's Hospices (2023). *How we help*. Available at: https://www.shootingstar.org.uk/how-we-help/ (Accessed: 29.01.2023).

Shooting Star Children's Hospices (2022). *A look inside dramatherapy*. Available at: https://www.shootingstar.org.uk/news/a-look-inside-dramatherapy/ (Accessed: 29. 31.2022).

Sinason, V. (1992). *Mental handicap and the human condition: New approaches from the Tavistock*. London: Free Association Books.

Stein, A., Dalton, L., Rapa, E., Bluebond-Langner, M., Hanington, L., Stein, K. F., Ziebland, S., Rochat, T., Harrop, E., Kelly, B., Bland, R., and Communication Expert Group (2019). Communication with children and adolescents about

the diagnosis of their own life-threatening condition. *Lancet*, 393(10176), pp. 1150–1163.
Sourkes, B. M. (2007). Armfuls of time: The psychological experience of the child with a life-threatening illness. *Medical Principles and Practices*, 16(1), pp. 37–41.
Testoni, I., Palazzo, L., Ronconi, L., Donna, S., Cottone, P. F., and Wieser, M. A. (2021). The hospice as a learning space: A death education intervention with a group of adolescents. *BMC Palliative Care*, 20, p. 54.
The Health and Care Professions Council (2023). *The standards of proficiency for arts therapists*. Available at: https://www.hcpc-uk.org/standards/standards-of-proficiency/arts-therapists/ (Accessed 09.01.2023).
Together for Short Lives (2022). *Categories of life-limiting conditions*. Available at: https://www.togetherforshortlives.org.uk/changing-lives/supporting-care-professionals/introduction-childrens-palliative-care/categories-of-life-limiting-conditions/ (Accessed 22.12.2022)

Chapter 4

Exploring the influence of multigenerational relationships on Taiwanese children through art therapy and object relations theory

Hsiao-Pin Lin, Tina Y. Chu, and Chien-Yueh Chiang

Introduction

Taiwan's culture is influenced by its geographical location east of mainland China, north of the Philippines, and south of Japan. While politically distinct from the People's Republic of China, the difference between the region's favoured name 'Taiwan' and its official name 'The Republic of China' reflects local and international tensions regarding Taiwanese identity, which includes indigenous cultures and an immigrant society from the past four hundred years, consisting of diverse ethnic groups[1] (Jiao, 2007; Yuan, 2014). These diverse communities value filial piety in which the elderly have absolute authority.[2]

In modern Taiwanese society, most parents in small families work, and grandparents often take responsibility for caring for their grandchildren. Intergenerational cohabitation is not exceptional in Taiwan (Hayslip and Kaminski, 2005; Hank and Buber, 2009; Sun and Jiang, 2017). It is common to encounter children growing up in a family structure of three generations living in the same household in the clinical practice of art therapists, a reality which can be attributed to Taiwan's long history of intergenerational cohabitation (Lin and Harwood, 2003; Chang and Chen, 2018).

The role of grandparents affects children in different degrees and forms. Clinical work, therefore, needs to focus on the relationship between the child and the parents and the grandparent-child relationship. This chapter presents three case vignettes of children engaged in art therapy in Taiwan. We discuss this therapeutic work from a psychoanalytic and object relations theory perspective to examine how the role of grandparents may influence the children and the parent-child relationship. Each vignette describes the family situation alongside the child's engagement and progress in art therapy. The first two vignettes (Moon and Lyn) detail longer-term work, while the third (Verne) describes a short-term, goal-focused, brief intervention. However, to set the scene, we briefly describe the context of art therapy in Taiwan.

DOI: 10.4324/9781003265610-5

Art therapy in Taiwan

Art Therapy in Taiwan began when Liona Lu, having trained as an art therapist in the United States, returned to Taiwan in 1989 to promote the profession actively. Following Taiwan's 1999 earthquake, Liona Lu became involved in the mental rehabilitation of traumatised children and families, and art therapy began attracting public attention. In the following years, art therapy became established in educational institutions, hospitals, and Non-Governmental Organisations. In Taiwan, only art therapists holding Taiwanese national counselling/clinical psychology licences are funded by national health insurance, while others work privately or are sponsored by charities. The art therapy practice of the authors of this chapter, Lin and Chiang, are supported by charities, while Chu is self-employed.

Multigenerational relationships: A sociological perspective

As the social and economic burden for young people increases, many younger generations rely on their parents to care for their children. In the United States, 24% of children have lived in a family of three generations before the age of five (Pilkauskas and Martinson, 2014). In the United Kingdom, the proportion of multigenerational family households has increased to nearly 7% of households containing two or more adult generations (Burgess and Muir, 2020). According to the Population and Housing Census Statistics of the Comptroller's Office of Taiwan (National Statistics, R.O.C Taiwan, 2020), there are 8.034 million households in Taiwan, of which the proportion of three generations living together accounts for 10.5%.

Multigenerational family structures have become a social phenomenon shared by the East and the West, attracting scholars to research and explore this from a range of perspectives. Hayslip et al. (2019) emphasise a positive evaluation of care provided by grandparents. Not only do they offer essential care for daily living, but also love and support. Grandparents become another attachment figure with whom children can discuss future directions; share emotions and feelings towards their parents or peers (Dolbin-MacNab and Keiley, 2009; Castillo et al., 2012); and provide protective social support (Dolbin-MacNab and Hayslip, 2014; Mendoza et al., 2020). In divorced families, parents rely on grandparents to care for their children when unavailable, regardless of whom custody of the children has been given (Ong and Quah, 2007). However, while grandparents positively influence grandchildren in many ways, Xu et al.'s (2022) systematic review of 42 studies across ten countries revealed that being brought up by grandparents had adverse effects on children's mental and behavioural health and educational outcomes in contrast to peers raised by biological parents. While some multigeneration research focuses on the inner strength of grandparents, including resilience, resourcefulness (Zauszniewski et al., 2013; Hayslip et al., 2014) and empowerment (Cox, 2008), the effects of stress on the grandparents' mental health of caring for their grandchildren and coping with ensuing behavioural problems relating to intergenerational upbringing is also recognised (Minkler et al., 1997; Sands and Goldberg-Glen, 2000; Poehlmann et al., 2008; Hayslip et al., 2014). Masten (2001) notes that resilience in human development arises from normal human adaptive processes in daily life. When grandparents rear their grandchildren, many of their grandparenting experiences support the development of resilience and positive adaptation in the lives of their grandchildren, which in turn reduces the grandparents' stress; promotes good physical and mental health; and ultimately supports the grandparents' well-being (Hayslip et al., 2014; Mendoza et al., 2020).

Taiwanese family relationships are based on filial piety, rooted in Confucianism. Filial piety is not only concerned with raising children but is central to all thinking about human moral behaviour within universal Chinese communities (Yang et al., 1989). Jordan (1998) suggests that the most salient feature of filial piety is respect and obedience to one's parents, including concern for their welfare. Filiality also extends to grandparents and all higher lineal ancestors. In many European countries, grandparents have few legal rights or obligations towards their grandchildren (Buchanan and Rotkirch, 2018). In many Western societies, the main social norm of contemporary grandparenting is 'being there' (Clarke and Roberts, 2004) or 'non-interference' (Harper and Ruicheva, 2010). Moreover, ageism has contributed to reducing the social status of grandparents in Western societies (Buchanan and Rotkirch, 2018). In contrast, in pursuing filial piety, the Chinese population bestows grandparents with a highly respected role of authority within the family and society (Buchanan and Rotkirch, 2018).

Indeed, data collected in Taiwan by Liu (1994) demonstrated that physical closeness among multigenerational family members enabled grandparents to take responsibility for childrearing. However, while the older generations may hold the ultimate power in decision making for childrearing and filiality in an agricultural or a fishing village (Chuang, 1981), in urban multigenerational families, young parents may conform less to the perception of filial piety than those in villages (Liu, 1994). Therefore, to maintain family harmony, parents and grandparents may reach a consensus on childrearing and filiality; however, potential conflicts between generations are latent (Liu, 1994).

Attachment and psychological effects of multigenerational household

Hayslip and Kaminski (2005) recognise that cohabitation with grandparents provides good alternative caring sources. When parents cannot provide adequate care, grandparents can safely and physically care for their grandchildren. For example, an Australian study noted that children raised by grandparents had appropriate levels of self-concept and emotional wellbeing (Downie et al., 2010); and according to Attar-Schwartz and Khoury-Kassabri (2016), emotional closeness to grandparents results in fewer emotional problems and increased rates of prosocial behaviour. However, in contrast, a study in the United States noted that children from households where the grandmother was the primary caregiver tended to have more externalising and internalising behaviour (Kelly et al., 2011), and a study in Thailand found that children reared by their grandparents were more likely to experience a developmental delay (Nanthamongkolchai et al., 2011).

While there is no research specifically exploring multigenerational family relationships from an object relations perspective, Poehlmann (2003) adopts an attachment perspective and suggests that when grandparents take on the responsibility of parenting grandchildren, three relationship processes simultaneously occur:

1 Disruptions in attachments potentially occur, especially in relationships involving parents.
2 Attachment relationships between grandchildren and grandparents develop or are revised.
3 Family members' internal working models of attachment and caregiving are challenged and shaped (Poehlmann, 2003, p. 149).

Object relations theory and multigenerational households

In object relations theory, the term 'object' does not refer to inanimate entities but significant others with whom an individual relates, usually one's mother, father, or primary caregiver. (Fairbairn, 1952; Hamilton, 1988). How a child's inner world is constructed depends on how the significant other responds to the child, whose relationships with others may vary and depend on different environmental factors. Children integrate experiences of their interaction with external objects and gradually form the inner self. Although the primary object plays a significant role in establishing children's interpersonal relations, others within the same family and the wider environment may also influence this process. However, studies of family dynamics from an object relations perspective on households complying with the principles of filial piety have yet to be found.

The following case vignettes will illustrate the relevance of these theoretical constructs for understanding the dynamics of art therapy practice with children growing up in intergenerational households.

Three case vignettes

Vignette 1: Moon

Moon was a nine-year-old girl from one of Taiwan's 16 indigenous tribes. She lived in a remote, mountainous township with her grandparents, father, and siblings. Moon's father had no steady job. When Moon was six years old, her mother left the family because of the father's long-term alcoholism and domestic violence, and she did not maintain contact with her children. Moon's paternal grandparents denounced the mother for fleeing the family home and indoctrinated the children into hating their mother and regarding her as a despicable woman. Moon was referred to art therapy by her schoolteacher due to emotional and behavioural problems and attended art therapy for 93 sessions over three years.

In Moon's first art therapy session, she presented with a smile, although the therapist was aware of Moon's need to keep her distance. She often had no preferences for the materials she wanted to use and would wander around them, remaining uncertain and anxious. At this stage, it appeared that Moon could neither connect with the materials nor bond with the art therapist. As art therapy continued, Moon became less anxious and began to explore her inner chaos through the art materials. However, her defences hindered any emotional self-awareness, her verbal expression remained flat, and any associations with her artwork remained at a concrete level, resisting any connection with her inner state. Finally, after six months, Moon included her absent mother in a dollhouse role-play, which the therapist understood as representing Moon's family dynamics. However, the role-play was rigid, and the plot was tedious. There was no interaction among the family members in what seemed to be a lifeless house, and Moon kept her distance from the therapist with apathy, uncertainty, and caution.

After a year of art therapy, there was a change in the dollhouse drama when the characters began to dialogue. A suicidal scene was played out in which the mother took the little girl who represented Moon and jumped off the house roof with her. After several suicidal acts, the little girl in the play finally screamed out, expressing her refusal to accept her mother's death and, in an enactment of self-blame, repeatedly committing suicide herself. No matter how often the therapist tried to rescue the little girl, she still 'died' each time, until in the last session before the winter vacation, Moon returned to an earlier scratch drawing (Figure 4.1), changed her smiling face into a sad one, then scratched off the figures of her mother, sister, and herself until there was nothing left. Collecting the black scrapings, she placed them in an origami box that she and the art therapist had made together. In this ritual-like process, repeatedly scraping off the black coating on the scratched paper and collecting the scrapings in a 'box of crumbs,' Moon finally revealed her deep sorrow, and her grief was contained in the context of the therapeutic relationship with the art therapist.

Moon expressed her feelings through creative and spoken language following this mourning process. In her use of the art materials, Moon seemed voracious; however, she began to care about her work and tell stories which reflected her feelings of loneliness, ugliness, and her unloved and forgotten self, now willing to connect in a relationship. In one session, Moon realised

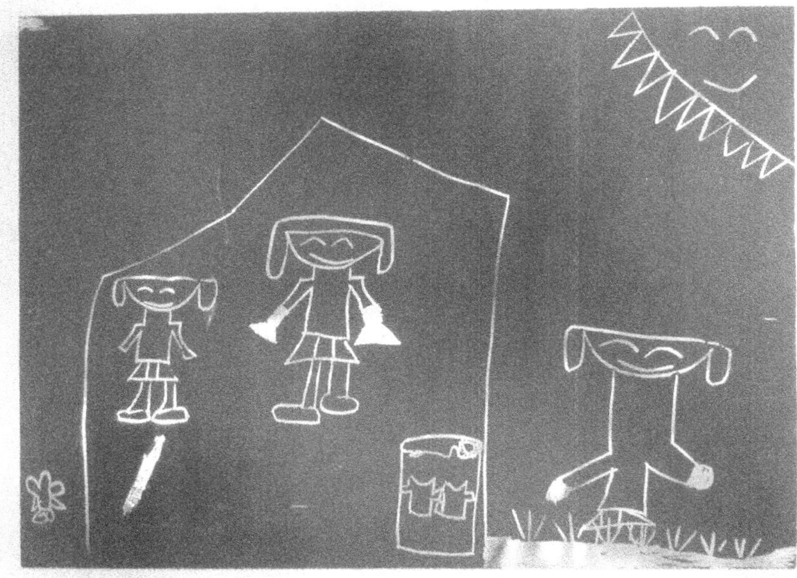

Figure 4.1 Moon's 'scratch drawing,' A4 black coated scraperboard with rainbow layer beneath.

that the difficult experiences she had been through were past injuries that had left emotional 'scars' just as the smeared paint had left marks on a mask that she had created in art therapy (Figure 4.2).

In another significant sequence from one of the art therapy sessions, Moon was able to finally acknowledge and take on board the reality of her family story: she took out the 'box of crumbs' in which she had collected the blackish particles scraped off her earlier scratch drawing, to represent her mother's ashes, and said, 'My mother is not dead. She escaped home after being beaten by my father, but she is no different from dead' (Figure 4.5).

In the following therapy sessions, Moon realised that her mother was not as despicable as her grandfather and father had portrayed and that the intolerable abuse in her parent's marriage had accounted for her mother leaving. Finally, Moon was able to accept her mother's decision to depart.

Vignette 2: Lyn

Lyn was five years old when she first received art therapy and was in art therapy for 39 sessions over 18 months. As an only child, she had lived with her mother and maternal grandparents after her birth, while her father lived

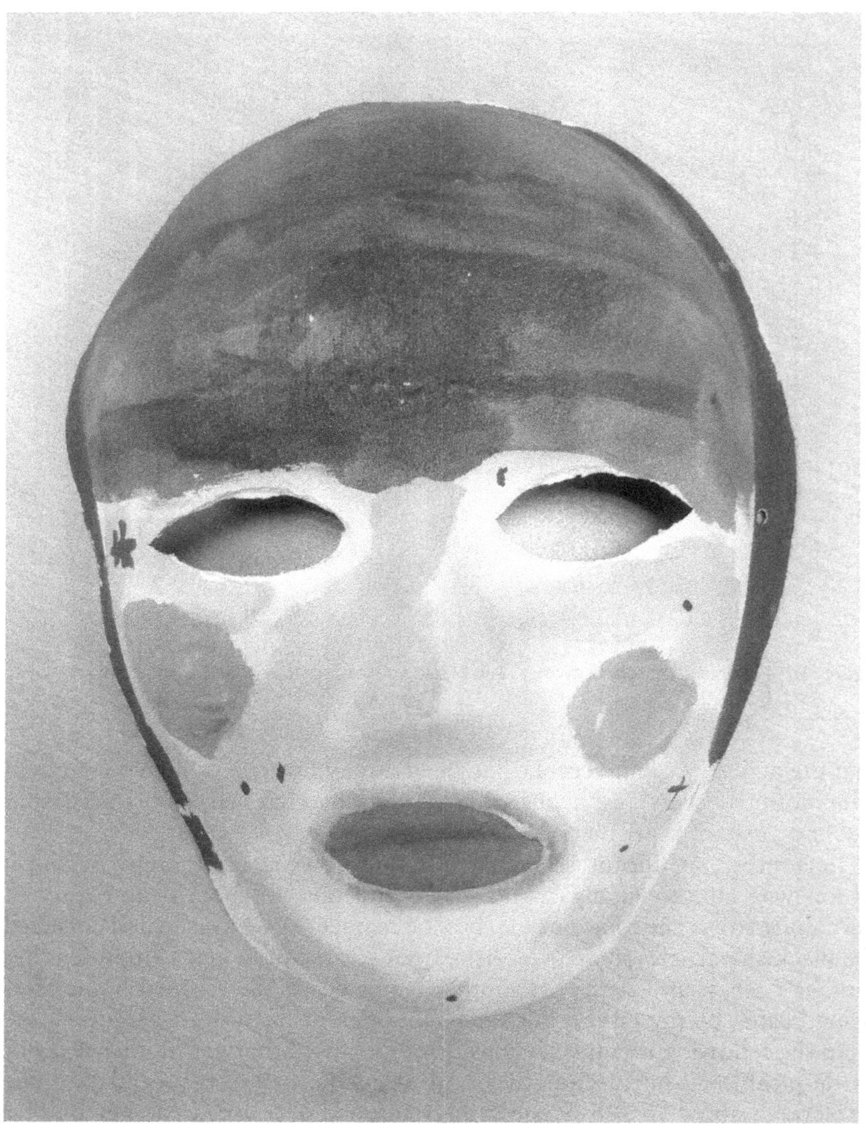

Figure 4.2 Moon's 'mask', prefabricated craft face mask painted with tempera.

in another city with her paternal grandparents. Following a divorce lawsuit, her parents agreed that Lyn could live with her mother and return to her father's house every weekend. However, one year after the divorce, Lyn's mother sought art therapy assistance as Lyn had developed separation anxiety and was demonstrating excessive anger. According to Lyn's mother, Lyn would have long emotional goodbyes with co-existing aggression towards her mother, who would often try to comfort her and accommodate her anger and anxiety. After the divorce, the grandparents from both sides of the family became resentful, blaming each other for the failure of Lyn's parents' marriage. As a result, Lyn became unwilling and often afraid to be near her father.

Lyn spent most of the art therapy sessions role-playing daily family routines. Although the plot changed as therapy progressed, the play's central theme remained abusive. Lyn consistently played and switched between two characters she had created in her imagination. First, enacting a mother who scolds her daughter with humiliating words and intentionally neglects her by depriving her of her basic physical needs of food, clothing, and shelter. Following this, the mother deliberately exhibits excessive love for the sibling of the neglected younger child and only shows callous cruelty to the other. Then, as verbal attacks in these scenarios gradually evolved into physical violence, Lyn created and played a second character of an abusive sister who secretly beats her baby sister after luring the mother away. As therapy progressed, the portrayal of neglect and abuse continued for several sessions until Lyn began playing doctor visits. The therapist was to play the doctor who prescribed glittered medicine packed by Lyn, who then began to care for and feed the previously abused baby sister doll.

Despite her reluctance to share her feelings initially, Lyn became more able to express her conflicting emotions, and her relationship with the therapist gradually appeared more genuine. Indeed, Lyn could now talk about her fears and express her love for her father. Significantly, she drew a picture with two doors, one leading to her father's house and one to her mother's house (Figure 4.3), and as such, accepted having two homes in her life.

In the final sessions, Lyn expressed sympathy for her mother and grief for her and her mother's difficulties during this challenging time. Lyn imagined bringing her mother to the art therapy room so they could cry together until the room was filled with tears and became a swimming pool where the two could swim.

Vignette 3: Verne

Verne, a 12-year-old boy, spent his early childhood in a multigenerational family where he was cared for by his grandmother while his parents worked. When he was six years old, Verne moved from his grandparent's house to live with his parents in a nearby neighbourhood but occasionally visited his grandmother's house after school. Verne was diagnosed with osteosarcoma[3] and admitted to the Department of Haematology and Oncology in a Children's Hospital for treatment, where his mother was his primary

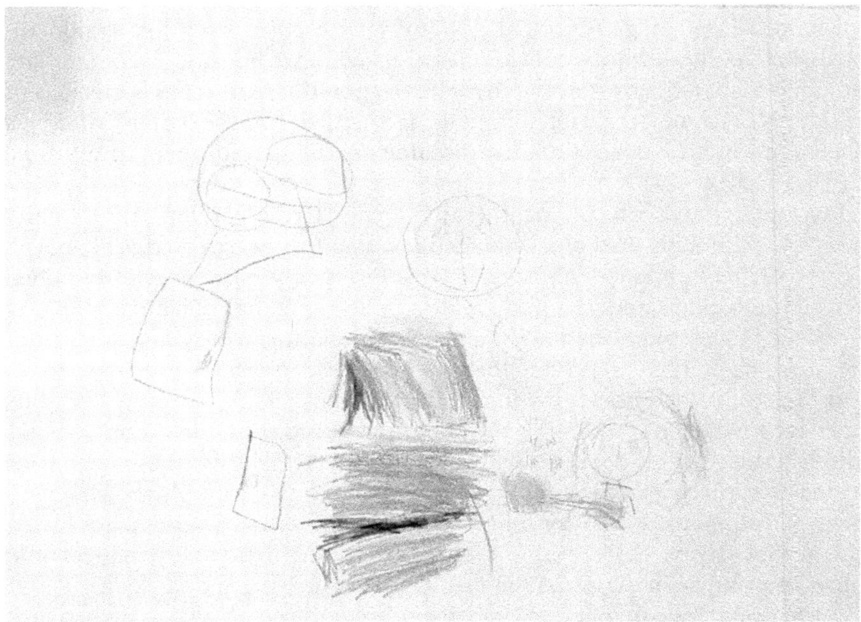

Figure 4.3 'Door to mum and dad', coloured pencil on paper.

caregiver. The medical team referred Verne to art therapy as he had become quiet and withdrawn during this difficult time.

Verne's art therapy sessions were short-term and goal-focused, involving six sessions. This brief therapy offered by the art therapist aimed to help Verne explore his feelings and connect him with positive life experiences to help him cope with his illness.

Verne showed his caring side in the first session and tended to suppress his feelings, as he did not want to worry his parents. However, tensions increased, and although he could not express these emotions verbally, he was willing to explore them creatively. With trust established, creativity and dialogue in the second session alleviated his anxiety-related breathing difficulties. This was the first time Verne had talked about his disease, his loneliness, of not being understood, his fear of losing his legs, and his inability to play basketball. Therapeutic work brought back memories of being with his grandmother, with whom he connected a positive experience of being supported through her empathy. Verne began to include Grandmother in his artwork. In one session, Verne started to cry, unable to speak. The therapist invited him to make art to express his indescribable feelings. Verne drew a line with two blue circles on two sides, himself on the right, his parents on the left, and a straight vertical line representing a wall between them. He

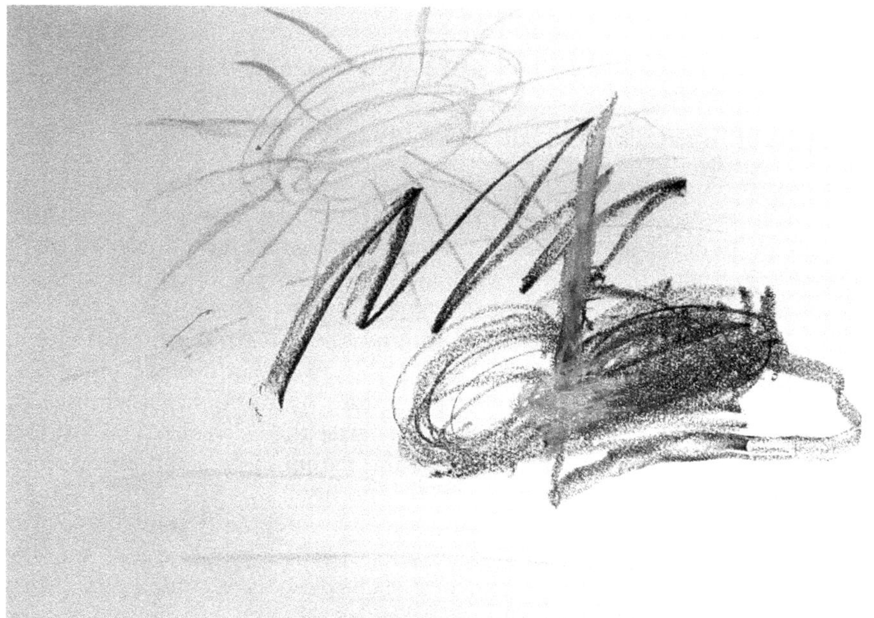

Figure 4.4 'Grandmother's warm sunbeams', oil pastel crayon on paper.

added red marks to this artwork representing his grandmother's warm hands. With this addition, this picture which had originally illustrated his loneliness now included a positive memory of someone he had felt secure with and to whom he could express his feelings. Grandmother's encouragement supported Verne like a sun warming his dark shut-off world, which appears in the drawing's background (Figure 4.4).

In his last session, just before he was transferred to another hospital, Verne created a scratch drawing of himself standing and smiling with his parents and his grandmother expressing the love and support he felt from his family during his illness. He added a heart on his chest and drew a bandage on his left leg with a bear face to represent the osteosarcoma on his knee. Finally, he drew himself holding a teddy bear (symbolising the tumour) and walking towards a warm home. These positive attachments will enable Verne to build his confidence and continue to cope with life's losses and unknowns in the future.

Discussion

Having explored some of the literature highlighting the sociological and psychological impact on children and grandparents of multigenerational relationships, we will now reflect on the three case vignettes and specifically consider disruptions in their attachment relationships, their relationship to the primary object, and finally, their capacity for symbol formation.

Disruptions in attachment relationships

According to Poehlmann's (2003) research on intergenerational childrearing, the grandparents' involvement may simultaneously disrupt and change attachment patterns in the family, strengthening the grandparents' role, while the parents' role may be weakened or dissolved. These findings are helpful in reflecting on the three case vignettes given above.

Lyn had lived since birth with her mother and maternal grandparents in the same household; her main attachment object was her mother. However, this changed as the grandparents on both sides of the family attempted to influence Lyn's feelings towards her parents after their divorce. This conflict appears to be the root of the tension in the parent-child relationship, particularly affecting Lyn's attachment to her mother.

When Moon's mother left the family, the paternal grandparents took over parenting responsibilities for Moon but negatively influenced Moon's attachment to her mother. In both these examples, the grandparents interfered with and hindered the mother-daughter attachment, changing the order of the grandparent-parent-grandchild relationship and the dynamic within the family in favour of placing the grandparents in the parental role.

Literature discussing the status and quality of the child's attachment to grandparents suggests grandparents can provide continuous, stable, physical and emotional care, meeting the criteria for forming healthy attachment bonds (Howes and Spieker, 2008; Li, 2013) In Verne's case, his grandmother became a stable attachment figure. However, according to Poehlmann (2003), this may disrupt the child's relationship with their parents (Sun and Jiang, 2017). Verne's strong, secure bond with his grandmother constituted his first attachment figure. Indeed, a good enough mother may not necessarily be the biological mother but someone who can respond to the baby's needs (Winnicott, 2005). When Verne moved from his grandparent's house to live with his parents at age six, his primary carers became his parents, and arguably his attachment to his grandmother was disrupted. It is important to acknowledge the sequential order of attachment relationships and to recognise that other relationships developed later in childhood will affect the first attachment relationship formed.

Disruptions of the relation to the primary object

While Lyn was an only child, the plot of her role-play involved the parents and two daughters, the latter constituting two contrasting representations of Lyn. In this way, Lyn's self was split into different characters: an older sister who was loved and a younger sister whom the mother abused. Lyn's object of interest was her mother, as her primary object, but her feelings for her were ambivalent, as the split between the two sisters in the role-play showed. However, her maternal grandparents, who lived and cared for Lyn, were excluded from the role-play. Interestingly, even though Moon represented her grandparents in her role-play, she portrayed them as characters for whom she had no affection. Instead, the mother, who was no longer present in her real life, frequently appeared as a figure of emotional significance in the play. Although Moon's early infant life was in a three-generation environment, her role-play indicated that she had established an early mother-infant relationship. The authoritarian grandparents could not replace the mother as the primary object for Moon.

Although Verne's grandmother was no longer his primary caregiver, he thought of her as someone who could emotionally support and reassure him. Indeed, observations from clinical practice suggest that Verne's grandmother served as his primary object rather than his mother. Verne's experiences of being contained by his grandmother in the early infant stage contributed to the development of object relations later in his childhood. They were sufficient to assist Verne in establishing object consistency (Hamilton, 1988) with the primary object. Despite the impact of significant illness, Verne managed his anxiety and fear with the support of art therapy, drawing on his inner resources of a good enough mother and a consistent primary object. The large representation of the sun in an orange crayon, which we may read as his grandmother's warming, benevolent presence, forms the backdrop of all other elements of the drawing, added later in blue and red crayons. These elements, representing Verne and his parents as close and yet separate, appear to be powerful; however, the marks representing the grandmother seem equally potent, if not more so.

Moon's mother fled domestic violence and left home. As Moon's grandparents influenced her towards hating her mother for what they framed as abandonment rather than an attempt to save her own life, Moon was unable to grieve the loss of her mother. As external objects, Moon's father and grandparents, rather than attuning to her feelings of loss, intrusively demanded that Moon both disparage and hate her mother. The same phenomenon is observed with Lyn, where grandparents, as external objects, attempted to convince Lyn to hate her father as the man who had disappointed them.

Influenced by family hierarchy and filial piety, these cases demonstrate how within the family dynamics, the grandparents' attempts to control their grandchildren can plunge the children into ambivalence toward their parents. During art therapy, Lyn eventually became aware of her love for her father, felt safe expressing these feelings, and accepted having two homes in her life. Having initially blamed and hated her mother, Moon realised and understood that her mother was not how the other adults portrayed her. Art therapy intervention helped both children regulate and integrate their internal conflicts. However, the therapeutic process involved in these transitions relies on understanding the child's capacity for symbol formation, which we explore in the following section.

The ability to form symbols

In the early stages of art therapy, Moon's understanding and experiences appeared quite superficial. Indeed, lacking curiosity and imagination, being incapable of abstract thinking, and presenting concrete attitudes are significant obstacles in therapy when, essentially, art psychotherapy aims to explore the symbolic meaning of each client's creation and play (Wadeson, 2010). Freud (1900) believed that imagination and the capacity for symbolisation were innate mental capacities, unconscious mechanisms for satisfying desire. Furthermore, the capacity for imagination and symbolisation supports the individual's ability to adapt to the frustrations of life and can compensate for what is lost in these experiences (Henzell and Dalley, 1984). These innate mental capacities belong to the primary process, where unconscious activity operates without regard for logic or reality. Freud indicated that concreteness results from defending against thoughts unacceptable to the conscious mind (Freud and Breuer, 1955). Moon's concrete attitude arose when her feelings of loss following her mother's disappearance became gradually repressed. This defensive mechanism impacted Moon's capacity for symbolisation in the early stages of therapy when she could not make much use of the art materials, and her connection to her work remained concrete and 'flat.'

Interestingly, Klein's (1930) seminal paper presents a case of similarly arrested symbol formation in Dick, a four-year-old boy diagnosed with childhood schizophrenia, although more likely now to be considered an autistic spectrum disorder. According to Klein's (2002) infant observation, the relationship between the infant and the mother from the beginning of life contains love, hate, anxiety, defence, and phantasy (Aguayo, 2002; Klein, 2002). In this way, the infant is full of ambivalence and aggressive phantasy towards the primary object and fears that any attack against the object would lead to retaliation in return. As a defence, the infant displaces the objective of their aggressive impulses to other less frightening alternative objects and begins to use symbols to alleviate internal anxiety and fear (Josephs, 1989). However, in Dick's case, Klein (1930) believed his aggression was too strong. The constitutional incapacity of the ego to tolerate anxiety had led to Dick's arrested capacity for symbol formation, and consequently, Dick's ego development was blocked. Moon similarly struggled with an arrested symbolisation in her early work but later would be far more capable of using the symbol in art therapy once she had begun to grasp the imaginary quality of symbol formation and its benefits and play and create more freely. We can understand this shift in Moon's work, considering that the long-term work gradually permitted her further development. It allowed her to become familiar with what Hinshelwood (2018; 2020), building on Segal (1978), calls the as-if function of symbolisation; as an ego function, it requires some degree of splitting of personality, which is both a denial of reality and an acceptance of reality. Hinshelwood (2020, p. 42) proposes that the as-if function of the ego is an 'integrated kind of splitting' of the personality, allowing reality and non-reality to exist simultaneously.

According to Hinshelwood, 'symbols depend on a tolerance of this dual attitude to reality, a "functional" conflict. The two sides of the conflict hold together, but they split apart in (...) disturbances of symbol formation.' (2020, p. 42)

In other words, when the ego must face conflicts and setbacks in life, the ego must choose between accepting reality and denying reality. The as-if function cleverly allows the mind to choose both, and the mind does not collapse as a result but helps the individual to accept and adapt to reality. Therefore, the as-if function is crucial for developing positive mental health.

Indeed, such an explanation can be observed in the play of Lyn and Moon. Lyn's abuse towards the therapist who role-played Lyn's sister (representing and symbolising Lyn's split-off 'bad' inner self) was a denial of reality. Lyn knew that it was only 'pretend' play. Still, when the therapist complied with Lyn's role-play, the scenario felt real to Lyn and evolved into an as-if scenario. This as-if function in symbolic play gradually helped Lyn integrate and accept her ambivalent feelings towards her inner self and her mother. As Urban and Koubová (2019) illuminate: 'At play the child continues to be the same person, however at the same time she plays "as if" she were a different person. Though she still experiences the same mother or father, she experiences her or him as a different one. This duplicity is explored through the child's own experiments,' which means 'testing her possibilities to act and receiving the responses from the world' (p. 179). In this way, Lyn slowly created a new understanding of reality that was no longer entirely dominated by her grandparents' denouncement of Lyn's mother.

Moon could not accept her mother's suicide in the dollhouse play, and the therapist understood the little girl's suicide as a form of self-destruction stemming from Moon's sense of guilt about her mother's departure. The suicidal plot appeared in the role-playing story 'as if' it happened. However, Moon did not die. This as-if function enabled Moon to follow a process of internal integration and to understand reality gradually. The repetitions and variations in this play held an important function, as Urban and Koubová (2019) explain: 'It is the repeated experience and experimentation with different forms of the "as if" which enables the person to perceive her potential and to test the surrounding world in a creative and critical manner.' (p. 182).

When Moon eventually took out the 'box of crumbs' (Figure 4.5) containing the scraped black particles, symbolising her mother's ashes, she said,

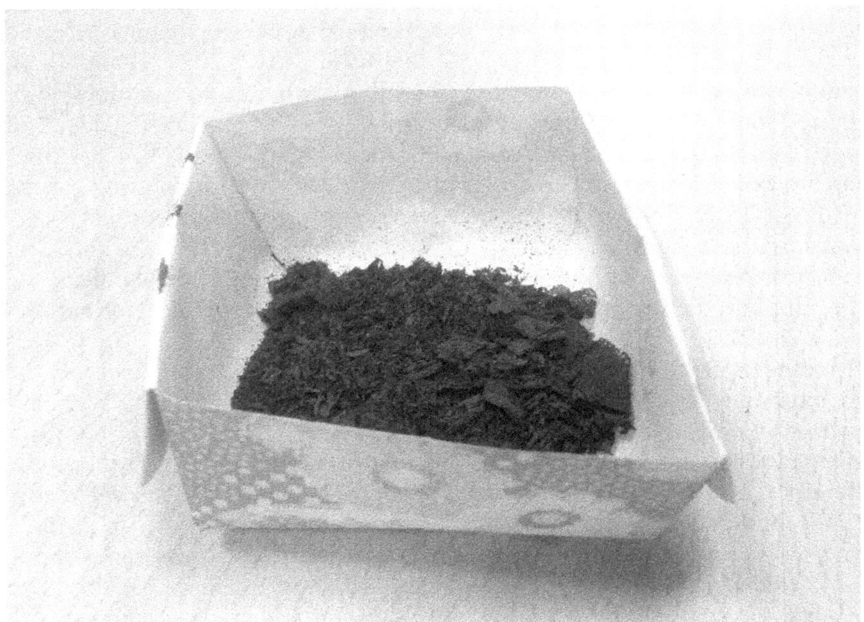

Figure 4.5 Moon's 'mother's ashes,' origami paper box with black scraperboard fragments.

'My mother is not dead. She escaped home after being beaten by my father, but she was no different from dead.' In this way, Moon symbolically enacted the disappearance of a past happy scene with her mother (Figure 4.1), whilst the origami box symbolised the containment of her grief within the therapeutic relationship. Hinshelwood's (2020) view helps us understand symbolic play's deeper modes of action during the therapeutic process.

While Moon's unpleasant life experience led her to distance herself from the therapist, the therapist kept and valued Moon's artwork, broken and meaningless as it may have appeared to be. Moon gradually became aware that the therapist had always accepted her regardless of her emotional state and had mirrored or responded to her with feedback. This containment, alongside the process of symbol formation, supported the cohesion of Moon's fragmented internal experience, enabling her to begin to take an interest in the therapist, respond to the therapist with affection, and develop her ability to symbolise.

Conclusion

The phenomenon of three generations sharing the same household is now common in many countries. It attracts research examining the advantages and disadvantages of living in multigenerational households from a range of perspectives. A consistent conclusion is that grandparents can meet basic daily needs and provide important physical care. Reflecting on our case vignettes considering Poehlmann's (2003) three relational processes, it is evident that when grandparents intervene in parenting or replace it, the relationship between the child and the primary caregiver is interrupted. This constellation changes the original grandparent-grandchild relationship and affects family members' attachment patterns. In addition, we argue supplementary to Poehlmann's (2003) view that it is not always the grandparents who alter the primary attachment between the grandchild and the parents, but it can also occur that a parent intervenes in the attachment relationship that the child has formed with the grandparents if they happened to be the primary caregiver.

From our case observations, we see a significant difference in response to loss from each child, determined by the quality of their object relations and the cultural presence of filial piety. As family patriarchs, grandparents maintain a respected authoritarian role, there are examples within our case vignettes of grandparents trying to influence their grandchild's attitude towards the loss caused by their parents' divorce. Furthermore, since filial piety is the central construct of family relationships in Taiwan, grandchildren are often forced to comply with this authority to maintain family harmony. Arguably, this strong cultural tradition increases the difficulty for clients in overcoming loss and other difficulties. Regarding the quality of object relations, it is irrelevant who the primary object is, but what is rather crucial is the intimate relationship between the primary object and the infant and the quality of the primary object's receptiveness and responsiveness.

In all three cases, we could witness how the children living in multigenerational families, to varying degrees, have used the art-making process to form symbols which helped them on their way come to terms with fraught family relationships, absence, separation, and loss.

These experiences reflect a consensus in the reviewed literature that the ability to symbolise constitutes a way to adapt to and build relationships in the real world. However, it has shown that studies looking at family dynamics in multigenerational households in filial piety societies are scarce from an object relations perspective. We hope this chapter provides insight into this area, contributes to the limited literature available, and encourages further investigations into this social phenomenon.

Notes

1 The indigenous Malay-Polynesians, the largest ethnic group before the Han people, immigrated and became the earliest primitive residents of Taiwan. They have lived on the island for thousands of years, and their language belongs to the Austronesian language family. The first wave of immigrants occurred in the late

Ming and early Qing Dynasties. Many Han people in China emigrated to Taiwan for asylum. Most were Minnan people from southern Fujian Province and Hakkas in eastern Guangdong Province. Many Minnan people married Austronesian women during the Qing Dynasty (1644–1912). The second significant immigration occurred in 1949. The government of the Republic of China moved to Taiwan due to the civil war, resulting in an influx of 1.2 million people from mainland China into Taiwan. Most of them were soldiers, civil servants, and teachers. Unlike early immigrants, these people come from all over the mainland, not only Han people but also from Mongolia, Tibet, and southwest China. Since the 1980s, new immigrants have arrived from China, Vietnam, Thailand, Indonesia, the Philippines, and other countries, nearly twice as many as indigenous people. Minnan people are the largest ethnic group in Taiwan, accounting for about 70% (Yuan, 2014).

2 According to Yeh and Yang (1989), the economic activities of traditional Chinese society are mainly agriculture, which depends on stable small-group collaboration. Family lineage has become the basic unit of operation in China's traditional culture and the core of economic and social life. Therefore, the family's protection, continuation, harmony, and unity have become important, leading to familism emphasising the importance of family. The younger generation must obey the elders, pass on their inheritance, and care for their parents. These concepts are called filial piety and constitute a societal ideology and practice strengthened in everyday life. Chinese society is deeply influenced by the ethical concept of filial piety in Confucianism, which originates in China. Although Confucianism has undergone historical changes, filial piety has prevailed in many morality and good deeds. Such thinking was brought to Taiwan with immigrants from China in different periods and strengthened and influenced the filial piety concept of Taiwan's original residents.

3 Osteosarcoma is a type of bone cancer that begins in the cells that form bones. Osteosarcoma is most often found in the long bones, more often the legs, but sometimes the arms, but it can start in any bone. Doctors select treatment options based on where the osteosarcoma starts, the size of the tumour, the type and grade of the osteosarcoma, and whether cancer has spread beyond the bone.

References

Aguayo, J. (2002). Reassessing the clinical affinity between Melanie Klein and Donald Woods Winnicott (1935–51): Klein's unpublished 'Notes on Baby' in historical context. *The International Journal of Psychoanalysis*, 83(5), pp. 1133–1152.

Attar-Schwartz, S., and Khoury-Kassabri, M. (2016). The moderating role of cultural affiliation in the link between emotional closeness to grandparents and adolescent adjustment difficulties and prosocial behavior. *American Journal of Orthopsychiatry, 86*(5), p. 564.

Buchanan, A., and Rotkirch, A. (2018). Twenty-first century grandparents: Global perspectives on changing roles and consequences. *Journal of the Academy of Social Sciences*, 13(2), pp. 131–144.

Burgess, G., and Muir, K. (2020). The increase in multigenerational households in the U.K.: The motivations for and experiences of multigenerational living. *Housing, Theory and Society*, 37(3), pp. 322–338.

Castillo, K., Henderson, C., North, L., Hayslip, B., and Smith, G. (2012). The relation between caregiving style, coping, benefit finding, grandchild symptoms, and caregiver adjustment among custodial grandparents. In J. B. Hayslip and G. C. Smith (Eds), *Resilient grandparent caregivers: A strengths-based perspective*. New York: Routledge, pp. 25–37.

Chang, C. O., and Chen, S. M. (2018). Dilemma of housing demand in Taiwan. *International Real Estate Review*, 21(3), pp. 397–418.

Chuang, Y. C. (1981). The Chinese family in a changing society: Case analysis of five families in Nan-Ts'un. *Bulletin of the Institute of Ethnology, Academia Sinica*, 52, pp. 1–3. (In Chinese with English abstract)

Clarke, L., and Roberts, C. (2004). *Grandparenthood: Its meaning and its contribution to older people's lives*. Sheffield: ESRC Growing Older Programme, University of Sheffield.

Cox, C. (2008). Empowerment as an intervention with grandparent caregivers. *Journal of Intergenerational Relationships*, 6(4), pp. 465–477.

Dolbin-MacNab, M. L., and Hayslip, J. B. (2014). Grandparents raising grandchildren. In J. A. Arditti (Ed), *Family problems: Stress, risk, and resilience*. Hoboken: Wiley-Blackwell, pp. 133–149.

Dolbin-MacNab, M. L., and Keiley, M. K. (2009). Navigating interdependence: How adolescents raised solely by grandparents experience their family relationships. *Family Relations*, 58(2), pp. 162–175.

Downie, J. M., Hay, D. A., Horner, B. J., Wichmann, H., and Hislop, A. L. (2010). Children living with their grandparents: Resilience and wellbeing. *International Journal of Social Welfare*, *19*(1), pp. 8–22.

Fairbairn, W. R. (1952). *Psychoanalytic studies of the personality*. London: Routledge.

Freud, S. (1900). The interpretation of dreams. In J. Strachey (Ed) (1959), *The standard edition of the complete psychological works of Sigmund Freud, Vols. 4–5*. London: Hogarth Press.

Freud, S., and Breuer, J. (1955). Studies on hysteria: 1893–1895. In J. Strachey (Ed) (1955), *The standard edition of the complete psychological works of Sigmund Freud, Vols.* 2. London: Hogarth Press.

Hamilton, N. G. (1988). *Self and others: Object relations theory in practice*. Lanham: Jason Aronson Book.

Hank, K., and Buber, I. (2009). Grandparents caring for their grandchildren: Findings from the 2004 survey of health, ageing, and retirement in Europe. *Journal of Family Issues*, 30(1), pp. 53–73.

Harper, S., and Ruicheva, I. (2010). Grandmothers as replacement parents and partners: The role of grandmotherhood in single parent families. *Journal of International Relationships*, 8(3), pp. 219–233.

Hayslip, J. B., and Kaminski, P. L. (2005). Grandparents raising their grandchildren: A review of the literature and suggestions for practice. *The Gerontologist*, 45(2), pp. 262–269.

Hayslip, J. B., Blumenthal, H., and Garner, A. (2014). Health and grandparent–grandchild well-being: One-year longitudinal findings for custodial grandfamilies. *Journal of Aging and Health*, 26(4), pp. 559–582.

Hayslip, J. B., Fruhauf, C. A., and Dolbin-MacNab, M. L. (2019). Grandparents raising grandchildren: What have we learned over the past decade?. *Gerontologist*, 59(3), pp. 152–163.

Henzell, J., and Dalley, T. (1984). Art, psychotherapy and symbol systems. In T. Dalley (Ed), *Art as therapy: An introduction to the use of art as a therapeutic technique*. London: Routledge, pp. 15–29.

Hinshelwood, R. (2018). Symbolic equation and symbolic representation: An appraisal of Hanna Segal's work. *British Journal of Psychotherapy*, 34(3), pp. 342–357.

Hinshelwood, R. (2020). The function of symbol-formation: Pinning down the ego function. *British Journal of Psychotherapy*, 36(1), pp. 32–44.

Howes, C., and Spieker, S. (2008). Attachment relationships in the context of multiple caregivers. In Cassidy, J. and Shaver, P. R. (Eds), *Handbook of attachment: Theory, research, and clinical applications*. New York: The Guilford Press, pp. 317–332.

Jiao, T. (2007). *The Neolithic of southeast China: Cultural transformation and regional interaction on the coast*. New York: Cambria Press.

Jordan, D. K. (1998). Filial piety in Taiwanese popular thought. In W. H. Slote and G. A. D. Vos (Eds), *Confucianism and the family*. New York: State University of New York Press, pp. 267–284.

Josephs, L. (1989). The world of the concrete: A comparative approach. *Contemporary Psychoanalysis*, 25(3), pp. 477–500.

Kelly, S. J., Whitley, D. M., and Campos, P. E. (2011). Behaviour problems in children raised by grandmothers: The role of caregiver distress, family resources, and the home environment. *Children and Youth Services Review*, *33*(11), pp. 2138–2145.

Klein, M. (1930). The importance of symbol-formation in the development of the ego. *International Journal of Psychoanalysis*, 11, pp. 24–39.

Klein, M. (2002). *Love, guilt, and reparation, and other works 1921–1945*. New York: Free Press.

Li, F. X. (2013). The influence of grandparent' child-caring on parent-child attachment relationship. *Journal of Ningxia Teachers University*, 34(3), pp. 130–133.

Lin, M. C., and Harwood, J. (2003). Accommodation predictors of grandparent–grandchild relational solidarity in Taiwan. *Journal of Social and Personal Relationships*, 20(4), pp. 537–563.

Liu, S. L. (1994). *Parental attitudes and expectations toward childrearing and filial piety: Harmony and conflict between two generations among Taiwanese families*. Amherst: University of Massachusetts Amherst.

Masten, A. S. (2001). Ordinary magic: Resilience processes in development. *American Psychologist*, 56(3), pp. 227–238.

Mendoza, A. N., Fruhauf, C. A., and MacPhee, D. (2020). Grandparent caregivers' resilience: Stress, support, and coping predict life satisfaction. *The International Journal of Aging and Human Development*, 91(1), pp. 3–20.

Minkler, M., Fuller-Thomson, E., Miller, D., and Driver, D. (1997). Depression in grandparents raising grandchildren: Results of a national longitudinal study. *Archives of Family Medicine*, 6(5), p. 445.

Nanthamongkolchai, S., Munsawaengsub, C., and Nanthamongkolchai, C. (2011). Influence of child rearing by grandparent on the development of children aged six to twelve years. *Journal of the Medical Association of Thailand*, *92*(3), p. 430.

National statistics, R.O.C (Taiwan). (2020). Summary analysis on 2020 population and housing census preliminary statistics. *Directorate-General of Budget, Accounting and*

Statistics, Executive Yuan. [online], [translated from Chinese website] Available at: https://www.stat.gov.tw/public/Attachment/1112143117MKFOK1MR.pdf pp. 21

Ong, D. S. L., and Quah, S. (2007). Grandparenting in divorced families. *Singapore Journal of Legal Studies*, pp. 25–50, July 2007.

Pilkauskas, N. V., and Martinson, M. L. (2014). Three-generation family households in early childhood: Comparisons between the United States, the United Kingdom, and Australia. *Demographic Research*, 30, pp. 1639–1652.

Poehlmann, J. (2003). An attachment perspective on grandparents raising their very young grandchildren: Implications for intervention and research. *Infant Mental Health Journal: Official Publication of the World Association for Infant Mental Health*, 24(2), pp. 149–173.

Poehlmann, J., Park, J., Bouffiou, L., Abrahams, J., Shlafer, R., and Hahn, E. (2008). Representations of family relationships in children living with custodial grandparents. *Attachment & Human Development*, 10(2), pp. 165–188.

Sands, R. G., and Goldberg-Glen, R. S. (2000). Factors associated with stress among grandparents raising their grandchildren. *Family Relations*, 49(1), pp. 97–105.

Segal, H. (1978). On symbolism. *International Journal of Psychoanalysis*, 59, pp. 315–319.

Sun, Y., and Jiang, N. (2017). The effect of grandparents' co-parenting on young children's personality and adaptation: Chinese three-generation families. *Asian Social Science*, 13(5), pp. 7–15.

Urban, P., and Koubová, A. (2019). Beyond the individualistic paradigm of the self with Donald Winnicott and Carol Gilligan. *Humana. Mente Journal of Philosophical Studies*, 2019, 36, 170–188.

Wadeson, H. (2010). *Art psychotherapy*. Hoboken: Wiley, pp. 3–8.

Winnicott, D. W. (2005). *Playing and reality*, 2nd edn. London and New York: Routledge.

Xu, Y., Wang, Y., McCarthy, L. P., Harrison, T., and Doherty, H. (2022). Mental/behavioural health and educational outcomes of grandchildren raised by custodial grandparents: A mixed methods systematic review. *Health & Social Care in the Community*, 30(6), pp. 2096–2127.

Yang, K. S., Yeh, K. H., and Huang, L. L. (1989). A social attitudinal analysis of Chinese filial piety: Conceptualization and assessment. *Bulletin of the Institute of Ethnology*, 56, pp. 171–227.

Yeh, K. H., and Yang, K. S. (1989). Cognitive structure and development of filial piety: Concepts and measurement. *Bulletin of the Institute of Ethnology*, 56, pp. 131–169.

Yuan, E. (2014). *The Republic of China yearbook 2014*. Taipei: Executive Yuan.

Zauszniewski, J. A., Musil, C. M., and Au, T.-y. A. (2013). Resourcefulness training for grandmothers: Feasibility and acceptability of two methods. *Issues in Mental Health Nursing*, 34(6), pp. 435–441.

Chapter 5

Music therapy as trauma-preventive social-ecological engagement in paediatric medical settings

A sounding of resources

Claire M. Ghetti

Solveig is a lively ten-year-old girl who loves skateboarding with her friends and taking her aunt's toy poodle for walks. She was recently transferred to the paediatric intensive care unit following an accident where she was hit by a car while walking to school. Solveig is recovering from a traumatic brain injury (TBI) and fracture of the femur of her right leg. Her parents are continuously present at Solveig's side and try to hide the anxiety and fear they feel. Could the injuries cause lasting effects? Torgeir, Solveig's nurse, notices the parents' distress and engages them in conversation as he checks on Solveig. His tone is upbeat and grounded, but inside he feels a weight—he has witnessed so many families in crisis.

When a child[1] is hospitalised, not only are the child and their[2] family impacted, but also all those in the contexts within which the child exists. A child's hospitalisation may be experienced as a void in the classroom, one fewer person in a tight-knit group of friends, the absence of a beloved niece to take the dog on a daily walk, or the recent addition of a distressed family on a hospital unit. Hospitalisation and treatment for severe and life-threatening illness do not impact a child as an isolated and independent being, but instead impact a child-in-context, and thus affect various aspects of the child's social ecology.

To understand how music therapy might play a role in promoting health across layers of a hospitalised child's social ecology, we need to take a step back and consider how we define health and how music relates to health. When health is defined from a socioecological perspective, it is understood not as a static attribute of individuals, but as a process nested in contexts (McLaren & Hawe, 2005). Health manifests in the multiple relationships between a person and their surroundings (Stige & Ærø, 2012). If health is understood as being relational in nature, then any one single frame, such as a medical or psychiatric understanding, has meaning but alone is not sufficient for understanding health (Stige & Ærø, 2012, p. 78).

DOI: 10.4324/9781003265610-6

When the modern profession of music therapy was first developed in Norwegian paediatric medical settings, it was done so with foundations in socioecological understandings of health. Music therapist and psychiatric nurse Trygve Aasgaard began pioneering work of muscialising the hospital environment as he developed music environmental therapy[3] in the mid-1990s (Aasgaard, 1999). Taking inspiration from sociology and social anthropology (Aasgaard, 2002), he understood that making music together was a natural means of social connection and health promotion (Aasgaard, 2004). Music therapy was understood as a process that promoted health by building from peoples' musical and social resources, rather than aiming exclusively on the reduction of symptoms and pathology. This chapter considers how music therapy can be a resource-oriented and health-promoting relational process while also being trauma-preventive for children, youth, and their families impacted by serious illness and hospitalisation. Theoretical and practical perspectives from pioneers of music therapy in Norwegian paediatric medical contexts will provide a foundation for exploring the socioecological potentials of music therapy.

Setting the stage

Among the Nordic countries, Norwegians were pioneers in establishing music therapy in paediatric medical settings from the mid-1990s onward (Ærø & Aasgaard, 2011) and have developed a broad presence in paediatric hospitals that is unique among these countries (Bonde, 2020).[4] Several aspects of the Norwegian welfare state have supported the development of music therapy in paediatric medical contexts and resonate with core family-centred practices in music therapy (Ullsten et al., 2020). Firstly, by law children under the age of 16 years have the right to have at least one parent present with them at all times in the hospital (Blichfeldt-Ærø, 2018; Pasient-og brukerrettighetsloven [Patient and user rights law], 1999). Generous family leave and sick leave policies make it possible to implement such laws, which means that family members are often present and available to engage in music therapy. In addition, children also have the right to be activated and educated during the course of their hospitalisation (Pasient-og brukerrettighetsloven [Patient and user rights law], 1999). Music therapy is mentioned specifically in national health guidelines for paediatric palliative care and for the follow-up of premature infants. For example, supported by research evidence, music therapy is mentioned in 'National Guidelines for Paediatric Palliative Care' (Helsedirektoratet, 2016) as a means for diversion, relaxation, and improving quality of life as part of a holistic approach to symptom relief. As specific recommendations for the provision of health care services, the national guidelines carry political and practical import.

With its social, ecological, and existential relevance, music therapy plays a unique role in promoting health within Norwegian paediatric hospital contexts. A shift in treatment philosophy in the medical disciplines to encompass more holistic, relational, and interdisciplinary thinking supports the presence of music therapy in Norwegian paediatric medical contexts (Ærø, 2016). For example, the importance of taking a holistic approach to care is evident in the national guidelines for paediatric palliative care, wherein music therapy is listed as part of a holistic, interdisciplinary approach to managing symptoms. Such thinking contributes to efforts like the development of 'advanced hospital at home,' where children with chronic and/or life-threatening illness receive 'inpatient' level care, but in the comfort and familiarity of their homes (Leinebø Steinhardt et al., 2021). Music therapists have researched pilot programming of music therapy as part of the advanced hospital at home interdisciplinary team. Findings suggest that music therapy can increase connection as a way to counter the isolation that can arise when such treatment occurs at home instead of the hospital, and provides a way to elaborate upon the child's and family's resources to enable vitalisation and foster joy (Leinebø Steinhardt et al., 2021). In sum, music therapy arises as a unique example of how the Norwegian health system can treat 'the whole person, including physical, psychological, and social needs' (Lindvall, 2017).

What is health?

Within a socioecological frame, health is understood as a relational concept, where health is constituted via relationships between the person and their surroundings (Stige & Ærø, 2012). Health is performed in ways influenced by culture and is socially constructed (Ruud, 1998; DeNora, 2000, 2007). For example, how we understand and respond to physical and mental states of being is mediated by social factors, culture, and aspects of our surroundings (DeNora, 2007, 2016). Thus, health is fluid and shifts over time, shaped by a person's individual biological features, but also by one's beliefs, behaviours, life circumstances, and social and physical environment (DeNora, 2016).

Socioecological understandings of health have origins in the ecological systems theory of psychologist Urie Bronfenbrenner (1979). Bronfenbrenner conceived of humans as developing in relation to the changing environments in which they grow, and that these environments are nested within formal and informal social contexts (Bronfenbrenner, 1977). The 'ecology of human development' then involves the transactions among the developing person and the nested social structures within which and in relation to which that person develops. The ecological environment consists of nested layers of micro- (relations between the person and the immediate setting, for example, school, family, or workplace), meso- (interrelations among the person's major settings, thus a 'system of microsystems'), exo- (formal and informal social structures that do not contain the person but influence the settings in which the person exists), and macrosystems (ideologies and other institutionalised patterns that exist in cultures and sub-cultures) (Bronfenbrenner, 1977, pp. 514–515). Ecological systems theory underpins socioecological models of health, as it helps explain how health arises through multiple nested relations among the layers of humans' ecology. Ecological thinking is crucial when considering health, including the work of music therapists in medical settings, as it demonstrates how working solely at the microsystems level is often not sufficient or is compromised by barriers at other levels (Stige, 2002).

Health can also be understood as including existential dimensions, where one experiences health by 'finding meaning and fulfilment by *being-in-the-world*' (Trondalen, 2016, p. 3, para 1). Children with serious illness can develop aspects of health and experience existential worth despite their illness (Ærø & Aasgaard, 2011; Noer, 2017). When health is understood as a relational concept, then it is possible to experience aspects of health at the same time as one experiences physical decline from a disease process. Thus, one's state of health is in active change throughout one's lifespan and can simultaneously contain both elements of 'health' and 'illness' as traditionally conceived (DeNora, 2016; Trondalen, 2016). Music therapy facilitates an important existential dimension as it provides a frame for people to be 'together in shared, wordless community where everyone can find room for their feelings' (Blichfeldt-Ærø & Leinebø, 2017, p. 46; author's translation). It is often not possible for music therapists to take away suffering, but they can create spaces where families are supported through their pain (Blichfeldt-Ærø & Leinebø, 2017), including support for existential suffering.

What is music?

Just as one can conceive of health as performative, so can music be understood as performative, reflecting all forms of using or making music (Stige, 2002). Like health, music may be understood as a form of embodied social practice and through such practice, health-promoting properties arise (DeNora, 2016). The health-promoting benefits that arise from engaging with music are thereby understood as naturally developing from the relationships music affords (DeNora, 2000, 2016; Stige, 2002).

Health musicking

Music is often conceived of as an object, and in the context of health, traditionally considered something that can be applied to promote some kind of desired outcome, such as relaxation or activation. Musicologist Christopher Small (1998) instead conceives of music as a verb, *musicking*, highlighting the multiple ways within which humans engage with music. Drawing upon Small's notion of musicking, along with social psychologist J. J. Gibson's (1958) concept of *affordance* and music sociologist Tia DeNora's (DeNora, 2000, 2007) considerations of *appropriation*, music therapist Brynjulf Stige articulated the concept of *health musicking*, as 'characterized by careful assessment and appropriation of the health affordances of arena, agenda, agents, activities, and artifacts' (Stige, 2002, p. 211). *Arenas* are the places in which musicking takes place, *agendas* the conscious or unconscious goals or aims, *agents* the humans involved, *activities* the forms of musical engagement, and *artifacts* the musical objects made or used (Stige, 2002). Music may afford us various forms of help or hindrance, depending upon how we appropriate it (DeNora, 2000, 2007). When musicking occurs in music therapy, it is health musicking and consists of 'the shared and performed establishment of relationships that may promote health' (Stige, 2002, p. 190). Music therapists aim to kindle capacities for health musicking (DeNora, 2007) that may be underacknowledged or underutilised among the children and families they engage with in medical contexts.

Even Ruud, a pioneer of music therapy and musicology in Norway, describes how musicking can be considered a cultural immunogen, wherein we express ourselves artistically and engage with cultural artifacts in a way that ultimately promotes health (Ruud, 2020). Our engagement in musicking may promote health through the four main 'musically induced antigens' of vitality, agency, connectivity, and meaning-making (Ruud, 2020, p. 3).

Health promotion in the hospital context

The care of patients and families in medical contexts is often dominated by attempts to treat and manage symptoms, while addressing underlying causes when possible. In contrast, the music therapist may focus on promoting health, via a type of *salutogenic healthwork*, for individuals, families, and the hospital milieu itself (Ærø & Aasgaard, 2011). Medical sociologist Aaron Antonovksy used his career to explore the origins of health (i.e., 'salutogenesis'), in contrast to the prevailing focus on pathology (Antonovsky, 1979, 1987). Through their work, music therapists explore the various ways that musicking contributes to health and serves as a resource during difficult life circumstances. A focus on resources underlines the resource-oriented approach to music therapy described by Randi Rolvsjord (2010). The sensitising concepts that constitute resource-oriented music therapy include the following: (a) focusing on resources, potentials, and strengths; (b) viewing the therapist/client(s) interaction as a collaboration, (c) acknowledging and attempting to understand the individual within their various contexts, and (d) understanding music as a resource (Rolvsjord, 2010, p. 74). Thus, music therapists may focus primarily on helping a child connect with inner resources and develop a sense of agency that helps them master the experience of hospitalisation, rather than primarily focusing on illness (Lindvall, 2017). It is often the case that in focusing on resources and potentials, the child and family are able to experience aspects of health that bring improvement in concrete symptoms as well. The overall goal is to promote health, regardless of what type of balance on resources or problems there is (Leinebø & Aasgaard, 2017).

Understanding the child in context

Developmental, familial, and cultural factors play a significant role in how children and youth experience illness and hospitalisation. Aspects related to emotional and cognitive development, previous experiences of hospitalisation and illness, previous experiences of pain, coping tendencies, and familial communication and coping tendencies all impact a child's ability to understand and adapt to their illness and hospitalisation (Reinfjell & Diseth, 2018). A child's developmental level impacts how they gain knowledge and how they understand their situation (Reinfjell & Diseth, 2018). It is important to remember that a child in the hospital is still a child, and as such, needs a sense of security, needs chances to draw upon strengths and continue their development, and needs to have positive experiences despite the associated struggles (Lindvall, 2017). In order to minimise the potential detrimental impact of illness and hospitalisation, it is important that typical developmental processes can continue during a period of illness (Gjems & Diseth, 2011).

By engaging in music making, children are able to connect with healthy aspects of themselves, providing a life-affirming link between their concept of self from home to hospital settings (Ayson, 2008). For most younger children, the ability to play and engage in fantasy is preserved and can serve as a resource when hospitalised. By engaging in musicking, a child can use music and metaphors to explore important themes without having to force such themes into adult-centric language (Noer, 2017). Through music therapy, children can approach challenging feelings and perceptions in a way that enables reframing and mastery (Ghetti & Whitehead-Pleaux, 2015).

As the family represents an important microsystem of the child's social ecology, the culture of the family is central when considering the ways in which children experience illness and hospitalisation. How a child relates to their caregivers and how the caregivers respond to the child's illness and hospitalisation directly impacts the child's experience of what is happening to them and how they experience health (Noer, 2017). Music therapist Marte Lie Noer describes that when a child is hospitalised, the family's 'wings are clipped' and the circles of movement and functioning are constricted (Noer, 2017). Like their hospitalised children, parents and siblings can also lose contact with their social networks and experience reduced opportunities for taking initiative (Noer, 2017). This creates a rationale for the need for music therapists to work at the mesosystem level, creating bridges between microsystems. Noer's context of work becomes the family and she aims to bring them into creative musical interaction in a way that supports their connection and resilience. Using music that is salient to the family's traditions and cultures (Edwards & Kennelly, 2011), or specifically 'song of kin' (Loewy, 2015) culturally-relevant parent-selected songs that are adapted to lullaby style and personalised to their infant, can help reinforce the connection between family members and help the child re-connect with healthy parts of their identity and home. Such connections can extend beyond family to include important social relationships within other microsystems of the child's social ecology.

Social-emotional engagement and belonging—A Norwegian perspective

Interdisciplinary staff members can be quick to notice how music therapy can serve as diversion for bored children or reduce symptoms like pain and anxiety, but the capacity to connect children and families to healthy identities and normal activities is underappreciated and less frequently noticed (Aasgaard, 2004). Music therapy may provide the means for a child to experience belonging and connection with others, even when physically separated due to isolation precautions or inability to come out of one's hospital room. Pioneering music therapists Stine Camilla Blichfeldt-Ærø and Tone Leinebø Steinhardt describe the example of Sonia, who cannot join the music therapy group that takes place in the large vestibule during shift change, due to fear of infection during palliative care for incurable cancer (Blichfeldt-Ærø & Leinebø, 2017). After the group has sung a few songs, a green thread is lowered down to the group from the third floor, and on the end is clipped a note with Sonia's wish for a song to be sung by the group. As her family pulls up the string again, and the group sings her chosen song, contact is established across the distance and music encompasses all who are present both near and far (Blichfeldt-Ærø & Leinebø, 2017). Through collaboration among Sonia, her family, and the music therapist, Sonia is able to make a meaningful contribution to the group and experience being a member of it despite the physical separation.

Connection to social network at home can also be facilitated through music therapy. Noer (2017) describes the use of 'Kråka' a black crow hand puppet, that provides a means for a hospitalised toddler to work through missing and being with (in fantasy) her older sister at home, experiencing connection and meaning through creative symbolic activity. During each family-centred music therapy session, the toddler musically rouses Kråka from its resting place and sends the bird on a mission, often revealing the toddler's own feelings and desires in the process. In such sessions, music therapy vitalises the family, expanding how they can be together, sharing good feelings, and experiencing meaningful moments that they perceive as being existentially significant (Noer, 2017). The various ways one can engage in musicking during music therapy can help families build tools for meaningful interactions, even towards the end-of-life (Leinebø Steinhardt et al., 2021). It can be salient and touching when parents are reminded of their child's vital and healthy sides, as they engage in musicking with support and adaptations from the music therapist (Blichfeldt-Ærø, 2018).

Normalisation and continuity

Solveig is recovering well but requires four weeks with her leg in traction to assure that her femur heals properly. The immobility is frustrating for Solveig, who is used to being very physically active, and she experiences some impulsivity and headaches that follow from the TBI. Solveig and her family have engaged in music therapy since their admission, first for providing stabilisation and orientation in the paediatric intensive care unit as she recovered from the acute stages of the TBI and then to help provide opportunities for social connection and mastery as she went through traction on the step-down unit. Solveig longs to join her friends in skateboarding again and works with the music therapist to create playlists of her favourite pop songs that her friends can use while at the skate park. Solveig sings along as they play through and assemble songs together. Due to being in traction, Solveig is not yet able to join the other children in the weekly music hour that occurs in the atrium of the paediatric hospital, but the music therapist arranges for two children of Solveig's age to come for a small group session afterward in Solveig's room. The three young people share a love of the same musicians, and this serves as an impetus for social engagement.

Music therapy provides an occasion for re-connecting with aspects of 'normal' life outside the hospital. Popular music may provide a means of connecting more personally with children, adolescents, and families and become a means of bringing 'normal culture' into the hospital experience (Blichfeldt-Ærø, 2018). The offer of music therapy services and relationship with the music therapist can provide a form of continuity of care that is rare in the hospital environment. Other disciplines may face practical restrictions that limit their interactions with families to one unit, while the music therapist can follow the child across units and levels of care (Blichfeldt-Ærø, 2018). Thus, the music therapist may play a unique role in facilitating a patient and family's transition and adjustment between units or levels of care (Leinebø & Aasgaard, 2017).

Communities of health

Since music is a medium that connects people and spreads through both space and time, it naturally becomes a way to promote the health of communities, including various communities within the medical setting. As music spreads through rooms, units, and sometimes across units via open atria, it offers a means to transform the hospital environment. The music therapist's task then becomes using music to 'humanise' the hospital community (Aasgaard, 2004, p. 148) through health musicking in all of its forms. Sometimes this takes the form of an interactive musical performance that incorporates staff, patients, and family and takes place in a more public area of the hospital. Other times, humanising through musicking may take place at a child's bedside, when the music therapist works in tandem with nurses or other staff and transforms the experience of routine care. What is most important is that musicking becomes a means of connecting, humanising, realising potentials, and creating possibilities. Seasonal musical celebrations, marking of special events, and weekly musical hours can create such occasions (Aasgaard, 2004). Aasgaard was a master of transforming parts of the hospital by muscialising them. He would lead the parade of patients, staff, volunteers, and visitors while wearing a top hat and playing a trombone, through the halls to a gathering place where they could enter a space of fantasy (Aasgaard, 2004). All of those who engaged would be treated as fellow musicians, and thus experience a transformation of identity (Aasgaard, 2004). Such extraordinary experiences can create a strong sense of fellowship and shared pleasure, an example of the anthropological concept 'communitas' (Turner, 2012). In such moments, where each person can play a musical part, whether singing, listening, playing instruments, choosing songs, or playing a certain character; children and families can display their resources, which otherwise might be overlooked (Trondalen, 2016; Lindvall, 2017; Leinebø Steinhardt et al., 2021).

It is worth mentioning that promoting the health of communities through musicking is not limited to the work of music therapists alone, as many types of music initiatives can support such efforts. Hospitals may form choirs or bands, in which staff from various professions have a chance to engage in music and creatively influence the environment and those in it. Volunteer musicians and special musical guests may also expand the options for musicking, and the music therapist can play an important role in building awareness of when such performances are beneficial and when they might become overwhelming for certain children or situations (Leinebø & Aasgaard, 2017). Thus, with their specialised competencies, music therapists may play a unique role in promoting health by working at the mesosystem level to support health musicking. It may also be appropriate for music therapists who work in medical settings to consider how their work could extend to exosystems and beyond, as they engage in initiatives that operate at the political and governmental level (Stige, 2002).

A focus on resources: Implications for trauma prevention

With the rationale for working relationally and in a resource-oriented manner well in mind, we now consider how the music therapist can simultaneously work in a trauma-preventive manner within medical contexts. Children can develop post-traumatic stress symptoms, post-traumatic stress disorder, and dissociative symptoms as a result of experiencing chronic or life-threatening illness and accompanying treatment (Diseth, 2006). Traumatic stress can arise from injuries requiring hospitalisation, from repeated painful or anxiety-producing procedures, or from the interaction of previous nonmedical trauma with current treatment and/or hospitalisation. Children who have experienced trauma earlier in life may have a resurgence of symptoms including hyperarousal, intrusive memories, and avoidant behaviours in reaction to hospitalisation and treatment (Saxe et al., 2003). A child's developmental level impacts how they understand and cope with what happens to them during hospitalisation. Younger children are particularly at risk for developing traumatic stress following hospitalisation for severe injury or illness; and across developmental levels, it is particularly important to manage pain in order to prevent later mental health consequences (Ziegler et al., 2005). Repeated painful procedures, lack of control, functional impairment, and restricted activity can all contribute to traumatic stress symptoms and increase the risk of long-term psychological, psychosocial, and familial challenges (Diseth, 2006).

Creatives arts therapies are particularly well-suited to prevent or ameliorate medical-related trauma as they provide opportunities for affect regulation and arousal reduction, sensory processing, externalisation, and attachment (Malchiodi, 2015). Music therapy provides a means for integration of somatic, physiological, and cognitive aspects of trauma responses and has particular relevance for doing so within medical contexts (Ghetti & Whitehead-Pleaux, 2015). If a child becomes traumatised during hospitalisation, important aims become reducing arousal, promoting stabilisation and managing pain, and avoiding pressuring the child to verbalise related to the traumatising experience (Gjems & Diseth, 2011). Music therapy is particularly helpful as it can bypass higher-level cognitive and language processing and provide in-the-moment focus and affect regulation (Behrens, 2011). Building from art therapist Cathy Malchiodi's (2012) principles of 'trauma-informed art therapy,' music therapist Gene Ann Behrens (2008, 2011) trauma-informed music therapy approach, and grounded in their own clinical and theoretical approaches, Ghetti and Whitehead-Pleaux (2015) articulated components of trauma-informed music therapy for hospitalised children and adolescents. Four of the nine elements are discussed here in light of the aforementioned discussions of health-promoting, resource- and socioecologically-oriented forms of music therapy to explore how such perspectives might also be trauma-preventive in a medical context.

Arousal reduction and affect regulation

A couple of weeks after her injury, Solveig began experiencing recurrent nightmares about the accident and developed high anxiety around the times of nursing care involving her leg. On some occasions of care, her heart would begin 'racing,' she would feel out of control, and she would attempt to push the nursing staff away. The music therapist met with Solveig and her father during a time when Solveig felt calm and the three tried out various breathing and focusing exercises, structured by live improvised music of

Solveig's choice. Together, they created a plan to use a specific breathing exercise prior to nursing care paired with a focusing chant during the nursing care, and a period of recorded music listening afterward. The music therapist was messaged by Solveig's nurse prior to her next wound care session, so that music therapy could start prior to the care to help Solveig regulate arousal and maintain a sense of control prior to and during the care. When Solveig became distressed during the care itself, the music therapist began their selected chant, coming into Solveig's line of vision and calmly but securely chanting, 'I'm with you, and you're with me. I can do this if I breathe' followed by a deep inhalation and slow exhalation. Solveig's father was present during the care and took over from the music therapist once Solveig was stabilised enough to follow the chants and breathing.

A common element across various models of trauma treatment is recognition of the importance of promoting affect regulation as a first stabilising step (Gjems & Diseth, 2011). Children who have been traumatised often experience elevated heart rate following traumatic stressors and sympathetic nervous system hyperarousal (Kirsch et al., 2011). Such physiological arousal occurs after triggering events, which may occur during nursing or medical care or in relation to noise, smells, or other sensory triggers. When a child is hyperaroused or has been triggered, the music therapist can use the stabilising rhythmic and temporal aspects of music to promote grounding and orienting to the 'here and now,' or sedative effects to reduce arousal (Ghetti & Whitehead-Pleaux, 2015).

The music therapist may work with family members to demonstrate how they can provide grounding and emotional support (Whitehead-Pleaux, 2013). Elements of proximity, tone of voice, simple musical or verbal cues, and sensitive use of touch can be modified to promote stabilisation and encourage the child's attention on the here and now. Any form of musical, verbal, or tactile support should be made in consideration of what types of stimulation trigger stress responses and the child's developmental, medical, social, and cultural background. The music therapist must also recognise that the parents and other family members may themselves be experiencing traumatic stress, and may need their own needs met before they can fully support their child (Loewy, 2016).

Depending upon how hyperaroused a child is, there are various approaches to musicking that can be taken. Live music carries the advantage that it can be modified in the moment in relation to a child's responses. Ideally, the child, family, and music therapist would have met prior to stressful procedures or treatments to identify the child's music preferences and coping preferences, as well as the child and family's culture, resources, and needs (Ghetti, 2012). When the child is hyperaroused, they may benefit from simple and direct instructions, a minimum of questions, and clear modelling of techniques (such as breathing exercises) from the therapist or parent (Ghetti & Whitehead-Pleaux, 2015). If recorded music is chosen, it should be selected with careful attention to the child's preferences, and consideration of sounds that might trigger trauma memories. Musical aspects of timbre, instrumentation, tempo, texture, novelty versus repetitiveness, and complexity are all important to consider when selecting music to reduce arousal (Ghetti & Whitehead-Pleaux, 2015). Depending upon the needs of the child and situation, musicking may consist of the therapist playing a grounding and steady strum on the guitar, while singing or speaking an orienting phrase (for example, 'We're here now,' 'Feel your feet on the ground'), engaging the child with a music-assisted relaxation experience with concrete cues for breathing or focus, or the caregiver singing a familiar and repetitive song while swaying to the beat with musical support from the therapist, among other approaches. Repetitive rhythm can harken back to being lulled by lullabies (Loewy, 2015; Noer, 2017). Parents are often an underutilised resource for supporting children in stressful medical situations, and supporting them in learning how to use their singing voice in a way adapted to the child's needs helps them connect with a pain management resource that is readily available (Ullsten et al., 2020).

Promotion of internal locus of control

A fundamental aspect of music therapy is that it offers opportunities for choice and control, which can support a child's autonomy (Robb, 2003; Leinebø & Aasgaard, 2017; Lindvall, 2017). When children exert choice and control within music therapy, it can reinstate a sense of internal locus of control, an important feature in trauma-informed care (Behrens, 2011). This value extends to the child's right to decline music therapy, when they might have limited ability to decline other aspects of care (Aasgaard, 2004). Deciding what they engage in during music therapy, what the music therapist does musically, and how they use music for coping can all contribute to a sense of control and feelings of mastery. In the case of medical procedures, when children are able to make stipulations to create a situation that is more manageable for them, they will have a greater feeling of control and experience more predictability (Gjems & Diseth, 2011). Children who experience repeated medical procedures over time may establish fixed rituals that help them cope constructively. The music therapist can play a role in educating other staff members in how they can support the child's coping strategies (Leinebø Steinhardt & Ghetti, 2020). Adapted ways of playing instruments and use of digital audio workstations can help make creation of music more accessible and thereby promote mastery. It is important that opportunities for choice and control are adjusted to the child's developmental level and level of arousal, in order to make them meaningful. Parents and other family members may be drawn into the musicking by the child making decisions about who will play, when, how, and what. In so doing, the child experiences a vital sense of 'doing' instead of 'being done to' (Rafieyan & Ries, 2007), which may be rare in the hospital context.

Promotion of healthy attachment and supportive relationships

Frequent medical treatments and prolonged hospitalisation can challenge familial and social connections. Children and parents can develop ways of communicating with each other that are shaped by periods of crisis. Musicking through music therapy provides an alternative medium through which family members can connect and relate, for example, through improvisation, family members can relate while letting go of intense dynamics that became ingrained during periods of crisis (Ghetti & Whitehead-Pleaux, 2015). Songwriting provides a way for families to appreciate the resources that each member brings, and to express deep emotions to each other. The normalisation and nurturing that occur during music therapy can support both children and other family members alike and can promote the experience of developmental gains. For example, a hospitalised infant may experience their parent as someone capable of comforting them and meeting their needs within music therapy sessions, that may contribute to the infant's development of secure attachment.

Integration of the trauma

The physical, functional, and emotional changes that accompany illness and injury can challenge one's sense of identity. A severe burn injury that impacts an adolescent's face, or injury or illness that results in a permanent reduction in mobility, will likely interrupt the adolescent's sense of independence and identity. Part of the work of coping with traumatic experiences is to learn how to integrate such experiences into one's expanded sense of self. Play, and the use of metaphors enable a chance to express, work through, and integrate contradictory experiences (Noer, 2017). Songwriting provides a particularly salient and personalised way to integrate difficult life experiences and periods into one's sense of self. In his doctoral dissertation, Aasgaard (2002) followed the 'life histories' of songs created by five young people with cancer. By tracing how, where, when, and by whom songs were generated, expanded upon and used, he was able to demonstrate how the songs connected the layers of each child's social ecology (Aasgaard, 2002). The songs facilitated expanded social roles for the young songwriters and provided a means of performing health for the songwriters and a culture of health for those in their surroundings (Aasgaard, 2002). One can understand this social-ecological connection as enabling a process of integration, a process that in itself is health generating.

Children and adolescents who have lived through life-threatening injuries or illnesses may need a tool for sharing their complex experiences with their peers and extended family upon return to school and home. A child may wish to create a song, musical slideshow, or music video that captures important aspects the child has gone through, and helps portray how the child has integrated these aspects into their current identity. Staff, family members, and locations in the hospital may be included, depending upon the child's wishes. Such a resource then serves to support the child's process of integrating traumatic experience, while it also provides a means for those outside of such experience to better understand the child's perspective. Some children may experience that it is easier to let such a personalised song, slideshow, or video tell their story than having to do so multiple times when trying to explain their situation. The combination of image, sound, and narrative can promote a deeply expressive process while also celebrating a child's integrated identity as they transition from hospital to home.

This concept of integration resonates with DeNora's (2007) considerations of how music affords individuals the opportunity to generate knowledge of the self, and within this process, to 'transcend difficult, stressful or extreme times and circumstances' (DeNora, 2007, p. 279). The process of integration, therefore, can be enabled by music's capacity to serve as a mirror and facilitate the generation of 'narratives of self' and thereby construction of identity that may support coping, rehabilitation, or transcendence (DeNora, 2007).

After three months in the hospital, Solveig was finally able to go home. She had experienced so much in such a short time and was surprised to find that she felt sad to leave the nurses, staff, and other patients she had grown close to. She was also apprehensive to go back to school and to interact with her friends, since her mobility was still compromised. She was glad to have the music video she had made with the music therapist. The video was like a trip through time and showed the ups and down she had experienced in the hospital, but most importantly it showed who she was, a resourceful young lady who found creative ways to master the challenges life handed her. She gave a copy of the video to her favourite nurse Torgeir, and eagerly looked forward to sharing a version with her friends.

Closing considerations

The complexity and pervasiveness of traumatic responses warrant a cohesive interdisciplinary approach. If a music therapist suspects that a child has become traumatised due to treatment, hospitalisation, injury, or re-activation of previous trauma, it is important that the therapist collaborate closely with the interdisciplinary staff. Psychologists can serve as important resources and support the efforts of direct-care staff (Gjems & Diseth, 2011).

Working with children and families who are undergoing or reliving traumatic experiences can be taxing for the music therapist. The process of musicking that occurs in music therapy may itself provide a means for a level of therapist self care. In music therapy, musicking consists of an experience of relating to oneself and others, as a promotion of well-being and a performance of identity (Trondalen, 2016). The music therapist then shares experiences with the child and family, which 'allows for recognition and partaking in one another's life at an existential level' (Trondalen, 2016, p. 7). Trondalen uses Yalom's (2001/2002) concept of 'fellow travellers' to underline that this relationship is joint, but is not identical. Thus, musicking can lead to an experience where not only child and family are vitalised, but also the music therapist and others who partake in the surrounding milieu (Trondalen, 2016). In any case, it is important that music therapist seek clinical supervision to support their growth and longevity in the face of this challenging work.

And finally, it is important to state that music is not always helpful. When music is used in ways that clash with listener preference, is inappropriate to the listener's current level of arousal, is associated with traumatic memories, or goes against cultural or religious beliefs, it may be ineffective at best and harmful at worst. In collaboration, the music therapist, child, and family find out together how music might be helpful to them, and it is important that this dialogue is open, honest, and considerate.

Conclusion

Children and youth who are hospitalised have complex histories that are shaped by developmental, social, and cultural factors. An awareness of how music therapy and musicking in general work on various ecological levels helps to expand our understandings of what is possible through health musicking. Health-promoting and trauma-preventing philosophies are not mutually exclusive and can be meaningfully integrated within the work of music therapists in medical settings.

Notes

1 'Child' is used in this chapter as a foreshortening of 'infant, child, and adolescent' unless otherwise specified, though the developmental and sociocultural differences between each must be acknowledged.
2 Non-binary pronouns are used in this chapter.
3 'Musikk-miljøterapi' in Norwegian (Aasgaard, 1999).
4 To date, music therapists provide services in five of six Norwegian university hospitals (Blichfeldt-Ærø and Leinebø, 2017).

References

Aasgaard, T. (1999). Music therapy as milieu in the hospice and paediatric oncology ward. In D. Aldridge (Ed), *Music therapy in palliative care. New voices*. London: Jessica Kingsley.

Aasgaard, T. (2002). *Song creations by children with cancer: Process and meaning* [Doctoral dissertation]. Aalborg Universitet. Denmark.

Aasgaard, T. (2004). A pied piper among white coats and infusion pumps: Community music therapy in a paediatric hospital setting. In M. Pavlicevic and G. Ansdell (Eds), *Community music therapy* (pp. 147–163). London and Philadelphia: Jessica Kingsley Publishers.

Antonovsky, A. (1979). *Health, stress, and coping*. San Francisco, California, Jossey-Bass.

Antonovsky, A. (1987). *Unraveling the mystery of health: How people manage stress and stay well*. San Francisco, California: Jossey-Bass.

Ayson, C. (2008). Child-parent wellbeing in a paediatric ward: The role of music therapy in supporting children and their parents facing the challenge of hospitalisation. *Voices: A World Forum for Music Therapy*, *8*(1). https://voices.no/index.php/voices/article/view/1796

Behrens, G. A. (2008). *Using music therapy to understand emotional needs of Palestinian children traumatized by war*. St. Louis, MO: American Music Therapy Association.

Behrens, G. A. (2011). Musiktherapie zur Behandlung von traumatischem Stress: Theorie und neueste Forschung [How recent research and theory on traumatic stress relates to music therapy]. *Musiktherapeutische Umschau*, *32*(1), 372–381.

Blichfeldt-Ærø, S. C. (2018). Musikkterapi i pediatri [Music therapy in pediatrics]. In T. Næss and A. T. Eggen (Eds), *Musikk på tvers, Råd-og tipsbok [Across music, Advice and tips book]* (pp. 97–102). Norway: Norsk Noteservice-Vigmostad & Bjørke.

Blichfeldt-Ærø, S. C., and Leinebø, T. L. (2017). Musikkterapi i palliasjon med barn - En støttespiller både for kropp og sjel, individ og miljø [Music therapy in palliation with children - A support for both body and soul, individual and environment]. *OMSORG Nordisk Tidsskrift for Palliativ Medisin [Nordic Journal for Palliative Medicine]*, *3*, 43–47.

Bonde, L. O. (2020). Music and health promotion in Danish/Nordic hospitals - who and how? An essay. In L. O. Bonde and K. Johansson (Eds), *Music in paediatric hospitals - Nordic perspectives* (pp. 149–169). Oslo: NMH Publications.

Bronfenbrenner, U. (1977). Toward an experimental ecology of human development. *American Psychologist*, *32*(7), 513–531.

Bronfenbrenner, U. (1979). *The ecology of human development. Experiments by nature and design*. Cambridge, Massachusetts, States: Harvard University Press.

DeNora, T. (2000). *Music in everyday life*. Cambridge, United Kingdom: Cambridge University Press.

DeNora, T. (2007). Health and music in everyday life - A theory of practice. *Psyke & Logos*, *28*(1), 271–287.

DeNora, T. (2016). *Music asylums: Wellbeing through music in everyday life*. London and New York: Routledge.

Diseth, T. H. (2006). Dissociation following traumatic medical treatment procedures in childhood: A longitudinal follow-up. *Development and Psychopathology*, *18*, 233–251. 10.1017/S0954579406060135

Edwards, J., and Kennelly, J. (2011). Music therapy for children in hospital care: A stress and coping framework for practice. In A. Meadows (Ed), *Developments in music therapy practice: Case study perspectives* (pp. 150–165). Barcelona Publishers.

Ghetti, C. M. (2012). Music therapy as procedural support for invasive medical procedures: Toward the development of music therapy theory. *Nordic Journal of Music Therapy*, *21*(1), 3–35. 10.1080/08098131.2011.571278

Ghetti, C. M., and Whitehead-Pleaux, A. (2015). Sounds of strength: Music therapy for hospitalized children at risk for traumatization. In C. Malchiodi (Ed), *Creative interventions with traumatized children* (2nd ed., pp. 324–341). New York: The Guilford Press.

Gibson, J. J. (1958). *The senses considered as perceptual systems*. Boston, United States: Houghton Mifflin.

Gjems, S., and Diseth, T. H. (2011). Forebygging og behandling av psykologiske traumer hos somatisk syke barn [Somatic illness and psychological trauma in children: Prevention and treatment strategies]. *Tidsskrift for Norsk Psykologforening [Journal of the Norwegian Psychological Association]*, *48*, 857–862.

Helsedirektoratet. (2016). *Nasjonal faglig retningslinje for palliasjon til barn og unge uavhengig diagnose [National professional guidelines for palliative care of children and youth regardless of diagnosis]*. Oslo: Helsedirektoratet. Retrieved from https://www.helsedirektoratet.no/retningslinjer/palliasjon-til-barn-og-unge

Kirsch, V., Wilhelm, F. H., and Goldbeck, L. (2011). Psychophysiological characterstics of PTSD in children and adolescents: A review of the literature. *Journal of Traumatic Stress*, *24*(2), 146–154.

Leinebø Steinhardt, T., and Ghetti, C. M. (2020). Resonance between theory and practice: Development of a theory-supported documentation tool for music therapy as procedural support within a biopsychosocial frame. In L. O. Bonde and K. Johansson (Eds), *Music in paediatric hospitals - Nordic perspectives* (pp. 109 –139). Oslo, Norway: NMH Publications.

Leinebø Steinhardt, T., Mortvedt, S., and Trondalen, G. (2021). Music therapy in the hospital-at-home: A practice for children in palliative care. *British Journal of Music Therapy*, *35*(2), 53–62. 10.1177/13594575211029109

Leinebø, T., and Aasgaard, T. (2017). Buildling musical bridges in paediatric hospital departments. In J. B. Strange, H. Odell-Miller and E. Richards (Eds), *Collaboration and assistance in music therapy practice: Roles, relationships, challenges* (pp. 285–303). London and Philadelphia: Jessica Kingsley Publishers.

Lindvall, M. (2017). Musikkterapi som helseressurs for barn på sykehus [Music therapy as health resource for children in the hospital]. *Tidsskrift for barnesykepleiere [Journal for pediatric nurses]*, 2. https://www.nsf.no/Content/3635048/cache=20172111214802/Musikkterapi%20Barnesykepleieren_04_17.pdf

Loewy, J. (2015). NICU music therapy: Song of kin as critical lullaby in research and practice. *Annals of the New York Academy of Sciences*, *1337*(1), 178–185. 10.1111/nyas.12648

Loewy, J. (2016). *First sounds: Rhythm, breath, lullaby trainer compendium*. New York: Satchnote Armstrong Press.

Malchiodi, C. (2012). Trauma-informed art therapy and sexual abuse in children. In P. Goodyear-Brown (Ed), *Handbook of child sexual abuse: Identification, assessment, and treatment* (pp. 341–354). New Jersey: United States.

Malchiodi, C. (Ed.). (2015). *Creative interventions with traumatized children* (2nd ed.). New York: The Guilford Press.

McLaren, L., and Hawe, P. (2005). Ecological perspectives in health research. *Journal of Epidemiological Community Health*, *59*, 6–14.

Noer, M. L. (2017). Kan kråka komme? [Can the crow come?]. In T. Næss and E. Ruud (Eds), *Musikkterapi i praksis [Music therapy in practice]* (Vol. 1, pp. 8–13). Oslo, Norway: NMH Publikasjoner [NMH Publications].

Pasient-og brukerrettighetsloven [Patient and user rights law]. (1999). *Lov om pasient- og brukerrettigheter [Law on patient and user rights]*. Retrieved from https://lovdata.no/dokument/NL/lov/1999-07-02–63#KAPITTEL_7

Rafieyan, R., and Ries, R. (2007). A description of the use of music therapy in consultation-liaison psychiatry. *Psychiatry*, *4*(1), 47–52.

Reinfjell, T., and Diseth, T. H. (2018). Pre-procedure evaluation and psychological screening of children and adolescents in pediatric clinics. In A. Guerrero, P. Lee and N. Skokauskas (Eds), *Pediatric consultation-liaison psychiatry* (pp. 193–215). Springer. 10.1007/978-3-319-89488-1_11

Robb, S. L. (2003). Designing music therapy interventions for hospitalized children and adolescents using a contextual support model of music therapy. *Music Therapy Perspectives*, *21*(1), 27–40. 10.1093/mtp/21.1.27

Rolvsjord, R. (2010). *Resource-oriented music therapy in mental health care*. Barcelona Publishers.

Ruud, E. (1998). *Music therapy: Improvisation, communication and culture*. Barcelona Publishers.

Ruud, E. (2020). *Toward a sociology of music therapy: Musicking as a cultural immunogen*. Barcelona Publishers.

Saxe, G., Vanderbilt, D., and Zuckerman, B. (2003). Traumatic stress in injured and ill children. *PTSD Research Quarterly*, *14*(2), 1–3.

Small, C. (1998). *Musicking. The Meanings of performing and listening*. Middletown, Connecticut: University Press.

Stige, B. (2002). *Culture-centered music therapy*. Barcelona Publishers.

Stige, B., and Ærø, L. E. (2012). *Invitation to community music therapy*. London and New York: Routledge.

Trondalen, G. (2016). Self-care in music therapy: The art of balancing. In J. Edwards (Ed), *The Oxford handbook of music therapy* (pp. 938–958). Oxford University Press. 10.1093/oxfordhb/9780199639755.013.19

Turner, E. (2012). *Communitas: The anthropology of collective joy*. Palgrave MacMillan.

Ullsten, A., Gaden, T. S., and Mangersnes, J. (2020). Development of family-centred care informing Nordic neonatal music therapy. In L. O. Bonde and K. Johansson (Eds), *Music in paediatric hospitals - Nordic perspectives* (pp. 1–25). Norwegian Academy of Music.

Whitehead-Pleaux, A. (2013). Pediatric burn care. In J. Bradt (Ed), *Guidelines for music therapy practice in pediatric care* (pp. 252–289). Barcelona Publishers.

Yalom, I. D. (2001/2002). *The gift of therapy. Reflections on being a therapist*. Herts., UK: Judy Piatkus Ltd.

Ziegler, M., Greenwald, M., DeGuzman, M., and Simon, H. (2005). Posttraumatic stress responses in children: Awareness and practice among a sample of pediatric emergency care providers. *Pediatrics*, *115*, 1261–1267. 10.1542/peds.2004-1217

Ærø, S. C. B. (2016). *Organisering av norsk musikkterapi i pediatri: En kvalitativ intervjuundersøkelse [Organization of Norwegian music therapy in pediatrics: A qualitative interview study]* [Master's thesis]. Norwegian Academy of Music.

Ærø, S. C. B., and Aasgaard, T. (2011). Musikkterapeut på en sykehusavdeling for barn: Helsefremmende arbeid for både pasient og miljø [Music therapist on a hospital unit for children: Health-promoting work for both patient and environment]. In *Musikk, helse, identitet [Music, health, identity]* (pp. 141–160). Oslo, Norway: NMH Publications.

Chapter 6

A DMT case study on child sexual abuse, trauma, and psychosis

Seeds of hope

Heidrun Panhofer and Maika Campo

Basque mythology is rich in characters and stories, and among them, although not so well known, is Martin-Txiki, little Martin. The tale takes place at a time when men and women did not possess seeds of wheat, precious goods that were controlled by giant guardians of the forest called Basajaun. *They lived in caves and sowed wheat on the slopes of the mountains and were feared by the people who craved the seeds but feared to approach them. One day Martin-Txiki put on huge boots and entered the woods of the* Basajaun, *defying their territory and boasting that he could jump further amongst their piles of wheat. Of course, in no time, the giants caught up with Martin-Txiki, who fell into the middle of a heap of wheat. When he recovered, he climbed out of the pile and ran home as fast as he could, his huge boots full of precious seeds. When he arrived at the village, he was able to offer the costly, cherished, treasured for precious Kernels, sows for seeds of wheat to his people.*

Introduction

Perhaps it seems a huge leap from the heroic Basque character to the protagonist of this chapter. This young offender had his first psychotic outbreak within the setting of an educational centre. Martin-Txiki, he who dared the giants, survived and stole a number of precious seeds for his people. Martin-Txiki is the name chosen for the protagonist of this chapter: a tale of deprivation, injustice, and enchantment, features that may sound familiar to those working with young psychotic patients.

No seeds, starving for the right nutrition. Martin-Txiki's parents would separate soon, and his biological father left his natal country Cameroon in order to find work in Spain. Martin-Txiki grew up with his mother, a stepfather and two younger siblings. A story of neglect and abuse, a small character that had no important role and remained unseen until he grew old enough to cause problems.

Martin-Txiki got to wear a pair of boots that were far too big when, at the age of fourteen, he was put onto a plane to join his father in Spain. He then was a boy who caused trouble, a boy who did not fit into his family. The biological father, who by then was living with a new partner, agreed to

DOI: 10.4324/9781003265610-7

take on his son in Spain. Forests and woods, new obstacles on the journey: the father kept moving towns because of his work and the fragile attachment with his new stepmother broke when she passed away. A period of going from one educational centre to another followed until Martin-Txiki ended up in a centre for young offenders, accused of having sexually abused a girl in one of the homes where he had lived.

Stones, troubles, a lot of aggression. Even in the penitentiary centre, Martin-Txiki was moved from one group to another, a last shift triggering his first psychotic episode. It must have felt like a moment of complete darkness, disorientation, and abandonment.

Lost in a deep dark wood, Martin-Txiki perceived a ray of light from somewhere. Voices from the past, his mother, and the Christian faith surrounding him in Cameroon blended with some ancient African rituals. Martin-Txiki grasped onto these specks of light and took off.

> *One night Martin-Txiki called his educator in the early hours of the morning. He could not sleep and could be heard talking incessantly from his room. When a companion opened his door, he was wearing a white robe, carrying a bible in his hands and repeatedly reciting a verse from the holy book. He barely slept that night, and when he woke up again, he could not get out of this loop where only the word of God could fit. This event triggered his first admission to psychiatry for several days* (Vignette extracted from the diary of the therapist).

Martin-Txiki's diagnosis of psychosis provided some explanation for his somewhat maladaptive behaviour. The image of a tiny boy with huge boots seemed just right, describing a human being who was wearing the wrong footwear to advance at his own pace in life, use his body in an efficient way and relate to others in a fluid, natural manner. The disembodiment of the self in mental health patients has been largely described by Fuchs (2005, 2016). Patients are not able to access the knowledge of their body anymore and lose their implicit way of working, including the pre-reflective way of 'being-in-the-world' that is mediated by the body:

> As the sense of self is bound up with the sense of others, disembodiment of self and disturbance of intercorporality mutually influence each other, resulting in a loss of natural self-evidence. A lack of tacit attunement to other people and situations (Fuchs and Schlimme, 2009, p. 572).

Similar to Martin-Txiki, he did not seem to possess a body that resonated and provided him with an intuitive comprehension of his own and others' emotions. From this split-off and broken place, the outlook on himself and the world seemed to be completely fragmented. He had lost a sense of how to deal with others and seemed more and more confused in his surroundings, caught up and trapped like the Martin-Txiki from the Basque mythology when he fell into the heap of grains, not knowing where he was anymore.

Recent research has shed new light on early adversity and psychological difficulties in later life (Schäfer and Fisher, 2011). The role of childhood trauma, especially sexual and physical abuse and, increasingly over the years, emotional abuse and neglect, has been uncovered steadily over the last decades. Whereas Post-Traumatic Stress Disorder can be detected in about 3% of the neurotic population, it correlates with 17–45% within the psychiatric population. Early life trauma can lead to lasting changes in the developing brain (Fan et al., 2008), and sexual abuse during infancy has been related specifically to hallucinations and delusions (Thompson et al., 2010).

At the time of Martin-Txiki's admission to the penitentiary centre, his story of abandonment, loss, and neglect was known to the authorities. The fact that he had been abused sexually over the years by his stepfather only emerged at a later point, disclosed by Marti-Txiki in a very lucid manner and, just like so many things in his life, completely out of context. His biological mother had probably failed to protect him from this painful experience, wiping out the particularly harmful relationship with the stepfather and endorsing thus Martin-Txiki's extremely fragmented and uncertain existence.

This constant ambivalence seemed quite evident when looking at Martin-Txiki's physicality. Clearly delimited, his body looked like a small version of a large armour. He was not very tall, but his muscles were well defined, fibrous, and seemed like a perfect machine for action. This machine worked completely disconnected from his head, leaving a dissociated, brisk body without limits. On other occasions, he would switch into a quite different mode, his eyes diving into passages of the bible while his body remained suspended and inert. In both cases, he seemed to have no limits, either going beyond his physicality in his automatic manner or not being able to stop his mind with his religious phantasies. His greatest fear was to go beyond his proper limits, nobody being able to contain him, acting with violence and a complete disconnection from what he was trying to overcome or prove, ruminating all the time.

Thus, one of the main goals for the work with Martin-Txiki was to provide a therapeutic setting that could offer some early holding functions and safe containment. The work with sexual abuse survivors through Dance Movement Therapy has been described by several scholars (for example, Cristobal, 2018; Goodill, 1987; Herman, 1997; Ho, 2015; Meekums, 1999; Pierce, 2014). Building on embodied perceptual practices, creativity, and expression, a stable relationship should help Martin-Txiki recapitulate some of his early relationships and mediate some of his traumatic experiences.

The relationship

Martin-Txiki responded with enthusiasm to the idea of receiving a therapeutic movement space with his tutor.[1] In some ways, this fitted in perfectly with his fantasy of being the chosen one, a recurrent religious dream that placed him in the position of saviour.

A classical DMT setting with a stable venue, place, and time was fixed, starting with a similar ritual and check-in that should help him to arrive in the present moment. However, from the beginning, Martin-Txiki would minimise his existence, either by confirming that he was fine and not in need of anything at all or tired, just wanting to sleep. Frequently he resorted to one of the passages of the bible in order to have 'something worth sharing'. He always found something bigger or more important than himself, and it was extremely hard to count on his presence.

> *During the warm-up, we worked on finding a safe place within the space, simply recognizing an area where he felt at ease and could build a basis to work from. My body served as a mirror, reflecting back some of his gestures and movements to offer him some reflection and presence in his existence. (…) My proposals kept changing according to his disposition, but on numerous occasions, Martin-Txiki wandered off into meditation, one of his many ways of avoiding movement. I started wondering if the movement and what moving with another person may involve would frighten him too much* (Vignette extracted from the diary of the therapist).

Relating to an adult or stretching out a hand to someone in order to receive help seemed an enormous struggle for Martin-Txiki. In his experience, similar to so many other survivors of sexual abuse, adults such as his mother or father or the surrounding community often had contributed to the experience of not being heard, and being silenced instead, experiencing secretiveness, betrayal of trust, fear and shame (Cristobal, 2018).

In her work with Martin-Txiki, his therapist found herself confronted with a frequent sense of feeling lost or losing herself, confirming Bennedettis's affirmation that 'in psychosis, transference often moves along paths different from neurosis' (1995, p. 60).

> *His speech had a point of lucidity that puzzled me. It was not at all vague, and I felt very clearly a need to stay alert and protect my own limits. At this point, I tried to differentiate myself, to make him feel the existence of a different other, although also available and respectful. I tried to take into account those feelings of mine as valuable information about what he might be feeling* (Vignette extracted from the diary of the therapist).

Working with a psychotic patient has been described as entering a room with many mirrors that can distort the reflections, send back multiple images, and confront with a mixture of uneasiness, fascination, and disorientation. Dealing with someone with a serious mental illness involves putting oneself in a relationship with someone else who sees their reality in a different way, with a different brain, but also with a body that moves in a different way, that interacts from another place, hardly understandable from a purely rational standpoint. Here DMT seems to have a lot to offer, allowing us to get to know the client through action. Through action, a shared process of co-creation of one's own world is sought while the patient transforms (Fischman, 2008).

At one stage, his therapist suggested that Martin-Txiki pay attention to his respiration, just breathing and becoming aware of how the air was flowing into his body and out again. As Hackney observed, 'Breathing is not only about connectivity but also our first experience of inner space' (1998, p. 64) observes. It thus seemed another way of connecting him with his own body as a container, a recipient that could take in and let go of the air around him.

> *During the eighth session, I proposed a very simple exercise that would help him recognise different parts of his body and later try to connect them. We did not get that far, but the first time he passed his hands in front of his face with closed eyes, he was able to feel the warmth of his own hands without touching his skin. All of a sudden, his eyes opened wide, he seemed deeply impressed, having been able to recognise his own warmth, his own body, a part of his existence. The fact that I was there with him, going along with his movement and witnessing this incredible moment of insight converted me into some kind of a magician* (Vignette extracted from the diary of the therapist).

Through the simple exercise of perceiving his own breath, he had in some way started to identify his own body, a body that had been numbed before, a body that had not existed previously but that he had now clearly felt through his own warmth, marking an important milestone in his existence. Samaritter (2021, p. 23) affirms that '(...) body and movement serve as the source and means of sensations, feelings, experiences, actions, and interactions but also integrate body organization and coordination in the therapeutic context'. The first step of recognizing his own physical existence and connecting it to his proper inner space had been undertaken.

> *Our warm-ups always started the same way. We kept travelling through the DMT space, myself accompanying him. Then we would find a place, oddly enough, it was always the same spot and ended up standing face to face* (Vignette extracted from the diary of the therapist, to be continued below).

In her study on survivors of child sexual abuse Ho (2015) puts a particular focus on the embodiment of the place and space concept. Building on attachment theory (Bowlby, 1989, 1999) which focuses on developing a safe base and a sense of security by internalising a secure relationship, an individual learns that the world is generally a safe place.

Because place and space can be perceived only through the body by seeing, sensing, feeling, and moving (reacting), the bodily experience becomes extremely important in helping abuse survivors to regain a healthy experience of place and space and thus in assisting them to recover a sense of security and freedom conducive to outward exploration (Ho, 2015, p. 10).

The study describes the importance of getting a sense of anchoring to a place, feeling the body in contact with a delimited surface in developing a sense of security and fostering healthy interpersonal relationships. Pierce (2014) confirms that for any healing to occur, therapy must necessarily begin with establishing a felt sense of safety within the relationship and developing skills for orienting to present time and space.

> *(...) I usually proposed to move each part of his body, starting from the feet and ending at the head, and he would follow me. All this meant passing through his body scheme, of being able to connect with each part, but also in an attempt to offer a relationship, a reflection that might help him to see the other in a more integrated way* (Vignette extracted from the diary of the therapist, continued from above).

The use of mirroring, kinaesthetic empathy, and nonverbal reflection have been described extensively as central DMT interventions with survivors (Campo and Panhofer, 2021; Koch and Harvey, 2012; Meekums, 1999; Pierce, 2014). Samaritter (2021, p. 62) confirms that dynamic movement experiences within the relational framework of a therapist-child interaction, as they are offered in DMT, may be particularly appropriate to advance a sensory-motor integration within a psycho-social context of the self-other relatedness.

However, since the moment Martin-Txiki had felt his own breath and with it a first notion of his existence, he converted his therapist into some kind of a magician, a mystical being with certain superpowers. His capacity to engage in symbolic play, a certain 'As-If'- function seemed to have disappeared, a quite common characteristic in schizophrenia that prevents the distinction between the factual and the fictional.

> This failure becomes manifest in the phenomena of *concretism* or a disturbance of metaphorical language; in *transitivism*, implying a loss of self-other boundaries; and finally in *delusion* as a breakdown of the 'as if' which until then marked the last connection of the patient to the intersubjective world. Now the co-constitution of a shared world fails and is replaced by the new, rigid coherence of delusion (Fuchs, 2018, p. 16).

This converts the illness also into an interpersonal disease that endangers the co-creative function of reality that our habitual interactions involve.

Similarly, Martin-Txiki either adored his therapist as a kind of magician or disappeared and resisted any profound engagement, connecting only when something seemed to be extraordinary and remarkable.

Weaving a skin

At one stage, the therapeutic work with Martin-Txiki became centred on his upcoming trial for the sexual abuse of another minor. It seemed as though he wanted to share his version of what had happened, and he was looking for his therapist's approval. Martin-Txiki chose to come back to the theme of looking for a safe space, and the need to cover himself seemed to become stronger and stronger.

> *He would lie down in a corner of the room, no matter if it was hot or cold, and wrap himself up, covering himself thoroughly, curled and rolled up so that, at times, I could only see his eyes. (...) He reminded me of a cocoon, and I was wondering if he was also preparing his transformation, waving his cover that would allow for his metamorphosis* (Vignette extracted from the diary of the therapist).

Anzieu (2016) argues that even the therapists' verbalisations if they come at the right moment and seem alive and accurate, may take on the function of a psychic envelope for the patient. Equivalent to a symbolic skin woven out of phonological and semantic planes, the words heard may allow the patient to reconstruct and ease the pain of the grievance.

Similarly, Martin-Txiki's therapist fed back with her physical and verbal reflections, attentive to his behaviour and as respectful as possible with his process.

> *Then he would ask me to always listen to the same piece of piano music and to lead a relaxation. Everything metaphorically seemed to configure that ball of silk thread that allows the caterpillar in nature to forget food and movement and concentrate on giving rise to the necessary metamorphosis* (Vignette extracted from the diary of the therapist).

Wrapping up Martin-Txiki with his preferred music or with gentle verbalisations could be compared to what Anzieu (2016, p. 72) calls creating the 'maternal environment', an outer envelope of messages that adjusts with a certain softness, leaving the space available in the inner envelope for the surface of the baby's body. That way, a place and instrument for the emission of its proper messages can develop: to be an 'I' is to feel the ability to emit signals that others receive. This tailored wrapping completes the process of individualisation.

> *Throughout the sessions, we changed that blanket for the elastic fabric, first reluctantly, because Martin-Txiki told me that he was cold and that the one I offered him was not enough. Over time lycra cloth became his first choice. It seemed more adapted to its own limits, it had the particularity of being able to define its shape in space. From there, I intervened, mobilising it in the distance, always respecting his space. Without invading his personal kinesphere, I was trying to figure out how to play with him. I stretched that elastic blanket and provided Martin-Txiki with many ways of making contact through the fabric. A tug of war marked our dance in several sessions, but I managed to get a smile of his more than once. I wondered whether he would ever be able to get out of his cocoon alone: If he seemed comfortable, why should he? To meet someone? He did not seem to have had nutritious experiences of encounters with 'the other' and after all, I too was going to disappear from his life* (Vignette extracted from the diary of the therapist).

Weaving a new skin seemed to be a leitmotiv throughout the work with Martin-Txiki. Establishing clearer body boundaries where others had invaded and vulnerated his existence represented one of the biggest challenges. At times, it would be an actual cover that was needed to wrap him up and create this protective place of change, other times, the limits of the space and the verbal or nonverbal reflections of the therapist would offer a safe and protective shield.

On certain occasions, the cover seemed to offer the possibility of separating himself from the outer world and his therapist.

> *When Martin-Txiki begins to use the blanket to cover himself, it feels like a barrier that he manages to put between us. He has used our moving space to hide, isolate himself, and remain immobile. I feel frustrated with these drastic changes, swinging from him having lots of energy and wanting to 'achieve wisdom' (because that was the objective that Martín Txiki raised when I asked what the space could serve us for when I introduced it to him) to him trying to merge with the ground, attempting almost to disappear.*
>
> *I feel that he could stay for hours under that cover, also contained by space and his classical piano music. Who needs my presence? … I am not clear if my presence actually makes a change. He has his refuge. Does it include me? But when I carefully lift one end of the cloth, the first thing I see is that his body reappears. His muscles are activated to try to hold the fabric, his gaze seeks me out to ask what is happening, and he verbalises and gestures allowing us to enter into a relationship. In addition, this moment of interaction becomes part of the ritual of several of our sessions. A part in which Martin-Txiki begins, at times, to play. The fabric seems to allow him an interaction from a safe distance, but the possibility*

of contact. It connects him with his own physicality in a different way from the body machine and close to one that plays in an intersubjective space (Vignette extracted from the diary of the therapist).

The vignette describes glimpses of a co-created space of interaction and play, moments of connection and mutual understanding. Hiding, being found, and not allowing the other to find oneself are quite common activities at the early stages of ego development. It seemed as though Martin-Txiki needed to repair many of these lost occasions of shared play and empathetic interaction. Kinaesthetic empathy, one of the key concepts of DMT (Koch and Fischman, 2011), seemed to provide the beginning of the healing for many years of neglect and abuse.

According to his needs, he used the blanket as a way to hide, disappear, or create a safe space, a cocoon-like wrapping which, perhaps at one point, would allow for his transformation.

Folie à deux

In the Basque mythological tale of Martin-Txiki, the main character boasts of being able to beat the giants when jumping over the heaps of seeds, a complete illusion that, for some reason or other, the *Basajaun* believe. How could they have been tricked so badly by the little boy? It seems as if both parts had engaged in something like a 'folie à deux', described as 'a very rare psychiatric syndrome in which a psychotic symptom is transmitted from one individual to another' (Vargas Alves Nunes et al., 2016, p. 339). Working with a young psychotic sexual offender certainly implies a central mindset, but believing in the supernatural powers of Martin-Txiki and the possibility of his recovery insinuates a different panorama. Indeed, the little boy falls into the heap, completely covered by the grains and unable to be rescued. Projecting a woven, new skin, a warm cocoon that might bring transformation, could be part of the distorted picture of a too bleak and unjust reality. Would his cocoon ever crack open and free a beautiful butterfly? Would the regular therapeutic work within an education centre for offenders allow for such a transformation? Would Martin-Txiki be able to get out of this heap of grains and manage to run home, saving some of the precious grains for his people? Was he the elected one?

Martin-Txiki's existence appeared distorted by his dreams, visions that seemed to have their proper life, even though they were not repetitive. Just like the heat of his hands that he had perceived, they had a magic and premonitory component, informing him about being 'the elected one'.

In his dreams, sudden movements of the universe were quite frequent: a huge crack in the earth that would open and wholes or waters that would cause a giant wave. Sometimes, all kinds of animals would arise from the earth, running away in fear. Then, another higher being would emerge, just like a God, always appearing serene and safe amid the greatest cataclysms. Martin-Txiki connected these dreams to moments where he had felt a physical presence around him, moments he had initially feared until he had connected them with those dreams of greatness. He had concluded that God had chosen him as the saviour, and those presences, like his dreams, were only signs of it.

Benedetti refers to hallucinations as 'not just a minus in psychotherapy, but a plus too. They do not correspond solely to a loss of reality but also to a gaining of a 'communicational surrealism' (1995, p. XVIII). At times, of course, it seemed difficult to work with this surrealism and, at the same time, keep in touch with reality.

> *During our third session, Martin-Txiki wanted to tell me what happened that night before he had been admitted for the first time to the psychiatric hospital. Someone had been with him in his room; he had clearly felt the presence of someone he feared terribly. He decided that he needed to leave the room and pray. His speech was confusing* (Vignette extracted from the diary of the therapist).
>
> *(...) There was a dream that, looking at it from a different perspective, seemed the original cataclysm. Sometimes he named it as such, but on one occasion; he presented it as a reality. Martin-Txiki told me that he had fornicated with the Devil when he was a child. And, most important of all, it was crucial to him whether I believed him or not. This episode confronted him with his uttermost fear, and somehow, he sought confirmation from me. All I could do was transmit to him that I was familiar with this incredible fear through him and that I felt the realness of the situation for him. His shared images, made up of particular and very rich alphabets, in which pain, stupor, and chaos could be clearly felt in the face of a heartbreaking situation that made possible a new way of focusing, seeing, and even feeling* (Vignette extracted from the diary of the therapist).

This dream could undoubtedly be related to the sexual abuse he had suffered during his childhood from his stepfather, but that had somehow converted the real person to a devil that kept haunting him in many ways. Trauma has long been known for inducing dissociative symptoms that affect an individual's inner anchors. Sexual trauma and the violation of interpersonal boundaries have particular relevance to these processes (Thomson et al., 2010). Benedetti (1995, p. 36) suggests that

> the appearance of cosmic hallucinations whose universality is not only a consequence of projections (to be understood as forms of defence) but rather are expressions of the tendency to perceive as parts of the world, which the self is unable to feel as its own.

Thomson et al. (2010) defend that the content of attenuated psychotic symptoms may provide insight into the underlying cognitive schemas of patients. In the case of Martin-Txiki, the hallucinations and premonitory dreams would seem to have found this functionality.

Benedetti (1995, p. 102) suggests that the therapist may start sending messages to the patient which are different from the psychotic ones, but messages of hope, of communication, of contact with the here and now. Indeed, there were moments of profound insight where Martin-Txiki questioned whether all this was connected with what he had gone through in his childhood. In many ways, it seemed a step forward in the relationship with his therapist when he stopped idealising her but recognised her as somebody different.

> *In the tenth session, when starting the check-in, Martin-Txiki told me he was depressed. First, he said 'because of you', then changed his statement to 'because of your words'. Faced with his recurring questions about my religious beliefs, I had told him previously that I was a different person with different beliefs. He then made several attempts to convert me to his faith but in vain. That day he seemed to accept me being different, even though he seemed to cover up for the loss of his magical therapist, telling me about a volunteer priest from whom he received visits. He claimed to be totally in tune with him and not with me. Martin Txiki ended the check-in by saying that relationships with other people transformed him, which surprised me and, in his case, seemed to be an incredible recognition of the other.*
>
> *We ended up talking about how human relationships make us feel different, and when engaging in movement, he identified his head as his most present part. However, he could not recognise any body part that seemed the least present. He wrote, 'I am satiated with answers, almost'. The session was exhausting for me, feeling that he would feel lost if I did not merge with him. I realise that I need to set my own limits with him while also having a strong presence* (Vignette extracted from the diary of the therapist).

The vignette seems to touch down on the sobering reality for both sides: A common illusion, a 'folie à deux' may offer incredible possibilities and fuel the dimension of hope and recovery. Martin-Txiki's only way out seemed to hang onto the dream of a divine figure who had chosen him as a saviour. He would also identify his therapist as a magic rescuer during one period. Being freed and safe could be a fantasy to trick away both sides from a far too bleak reality of abuse and injustice, of a life-long diagnostic of psychosis and a long prison sentence for abusing yet another youngster.

Conclusions

This book chapter weaves a red thread between early childhood trauma and psychosis, narrating the story of Martin-Txiki, a young offender who had his first psychotic episode in a centre for offenders.

> The evidence for an association between childhood trauma and psychosis is steadily accumulating. 'More research is (...) needed to develop further and evaluate appropriate treatments for psychotic patients suffering from the consequences of childhood trauma. Nevertheless, the existing trials suggest that patients with psychotic disorders can benefit from both present-focused and trauma-focused treatments' (Schäfer and Fisher, 2011, p. 365).

DMT offers a present-focused approach as it works with the body and all bodily movement, always drawing the patient back to the present moment through action. Psychosis is characterised by a fragmented, split-off way of experiencing the body. The extreme disembodiment of the self and disturbance has far-reaching effects on dealing with others, an important factor tackled effectively by the dynamic movement experiences within an intercorporeal framework, always present in the DMT.

As described by other authors from the field (Ho, 2015; Pierce, 2014), the re-building of a secure base, a safe place from where to explore, presents the first part of the work with survivors of sexual abuse as anchoring the body in a safe space within a secure relationship is a necessary basis for further healing. DMT interventions such as mirroring, kinaesthetic empathy, and nonverbal reflection have been described extensively as central DMT interventions with survivors (Campo and Panhofer, 2021; Koch and Harvey, 2012; Meekums, 1999; Pierce, 2014). Some early relationships can be recapitulated within the relational framework of a therapist-client interaction, and traumatic experiences may be mediated in movement (Campo and Panhofer, 2021). Martin-Txiki's story is yet another tale without a happy ending. It points at an unspoken injustice, a vicious circle of far too high numbers of sexual abuse and trauma in early childhood.

The Martin-Txiki from the Basque mythology escapes, saving some precious seeds for himself and his community. The story of the young boy from Cameroon who, as this chapter draws to an end, is still held in a centre for young offenders is yet to be continued.

Note

1 The second author of the chapter, Maika Campo, was Martin-Txiki's therapist.

References

Anzieu, D. (2016). *El yo piel*. Madrid: Editorial Biblioteca Nueva, S.L.

Benedetti, G. (1995). *Psychotherapy of schizophrenia*. New Jersey: Editorial Aronson.

Bowlby, J. (1989). *Una base segura. Aplicaciones clínicas de una teoría del apego*. Barcelona: Editorial Paidós Ibérica S.A.

Bowlby, J. (1999). *Attachment and loss* (Vol. 1). New York: Basic Books.

Campo, M., and Panhofer, H. (2021). How Pippo got to drive a fast car. In Uwe Herrmann, Margaret Hills de Zarate and Salvo Pitruzzella (Eds), *Arts therapies and the mental health of children and Young people*. (Vol. 1). London: Routledge.

Cristobal, K. A. (2018). Power of touch: Working with survivors of sexual abuse within dance/movement therapy. *American Journal for Dance Therapy*, 40, pp. 68–86. 10.1007/s10465-018-9275-7.

Fan, X., Henderson, D. C., Nguyen, D. D., Cather, C., Freudenreich, O., Eden-Evins, A., Borba, C. P., and Goff, D. C. (2008). Posttraumatic stress disorder, cognitive function and quality of life in patients with schizophrenia. *Psychiatry Research*, 1 (59), pp. 140–146. 10.1016/j.psychres.2007.10.012.

Fischman, D. (2008). Relación terapéutica y empatía kinestésica. In H. Wengrower and S. Chaiklin (Eds), *La vida es danza*. Barcelona: Gedisa, pp. 81–96.

Fuchs, T. (2005). *Corporealised and disembodied minds a phenomenological view of the body in melancholia and schizophrenia*. Project Muse: The Johns Hopkins University Press.

Fuchs, T., and Schlimme, J. E. (2009). Embodiment and psychopathology: A phenomenological perspective. *Current Opinion in Psychiatry*, 22(6), pp. 570–575. 10.1097/YCO.0B013E3283318E5C

Fuchs, T. (2016). Intercorporality and Interaffectivity. *Phenomenology and Mind*, 11, pp. 194–209.

Fuchs, T. (2018). The human 'as-if '-function and its loss in schizophrenia. Retrieved from https://dsc.duq.edu/phenomenologysymposium/17.

Goodill, S. W. (1987). Dance/movement therapy with abused children. *The Arts in Psychotherapy*, 14, pp. 59–68.

Hackney, P. (1998). *Making connections: Total body integration through Bartenieff fundamentals*. Amsterdam: Gordon and Breach.

Herman, L. (1997). Good enough fairy tales for resolving sexual abuse trauma. *The Arts in Psychotherapy*, 24(5), pp. 439–445.

Ho, R. T. (2015). A place and space to survive: A dance/movement therapy program for childhood sexual abuse survivors. *The Arts in Psychotherapy*, 46, pp. 9–16.

Koch, S. C., and Harvey, S. (2012). Dance/movement therapy with traumatised dissociative patients. In S. C. Koch, T. Fuchs, M. Summa, C. Müller (Eds), *Body memory, metaphor and movement*. Amsterdam: John Benjamin, pp. 369–385.

Koch, S., and Fischman, D. (2011). Embodied enactive dance/movement therapy. *American Journal of Dance Therapy*, 33, pp. 57–72. 10.1007/s10465-011-9108-4.

Meekums, B. (1999). A creative model for recovery from child sexual abuse trauma. *The Arts in Psychotherapy*, 26(4), pp. 247–259. 10.1016/S0197-4556(98)00076-8.

Pierce, L. (2014). The integrative power of dance/movement therapy: Implications for the treatment of dissociation and developmental trauma. *The Arts in Psychotherapy*, 41(1), pp. 7–15. 10.1016/j.aip.2013.10.002.

Samaritter, R. (2021). Dance movement therapy with children and adolescents. In S. Pitruzzella, M. Hills de Zarate, and Uwe Herrmann (Eds), *Arts therapies and the mental health of children and young people*. London: Routledge, pp. 60–70.

Schäfer, I. and Fisher, H. L. (2011). Childhood trauma and psychosis – What is the evidence? *Dialogues in Clinical Neuroscience*, 13(3), pp. 360–365.

Thompson, A., Nelson, B., McNab, C., Simmons, M., Leicester, S., McGorry, P. D., Bechdolf, A., and Yung, A. (2010). Psychotic symptoms with sexual content in the "ultra high risk" for psychosis population: Frequency and association with sexual trauma. *Psychiatry Research*, 177, pp. 84–91.

Vargas Alves Nunes, A., Odebrecht Vargas, S., Strano, T., Pascolat, S., Schier Doria, G., and Nasser Ehlke, Mr. (2016). Folie à deux and its interaction with early life stress: A case report. *Journal of Medical Case Reports*, 10, p. 339. 10.1186/s13256-016-1128-8.

Chapter 7

Arts therapies and psychoeducation for adolescents in India

Project Reflect

Preetha Ramasubramanian and Anshuma Kshetrapal

Introduction

While training in the UK, both authors experienced a fixed and reliable context. The various guidelines and ethics compliance documents were support systems that they could refer to when needed. However, returning to India, they found that there was no licensure board for Arts Therapists and no culturally relevant ethics documents that could guide them. There was also a lack of supervision, follow-up to check the effectiveness of training of primary care workers in mental health, funding, and resources. These factors posed a challenge to integrating classical mental health services with health care in any setting (Mahajan et al., 2019).

During a conference presentation in 2016, both authors found themselves discussing similar experiences and ethical dilemmas. Their struggle to maintain their ethical position brought them together despite their cultural differences, as Anshuma is from North India and Preetha from South India. They both felt unsupported systemically and over several meetings, they realised that they had taken similar routes to adapt to their cultural contexts and constraints. Thus began a journey of peer supervision and discussions around developing an ecosystem through endeavours best suited to develop the field of Arts Therapies in India. Project Reflect was the first of such endeavours. Since both authors worked in systems that produced common issues, they identified the necessity for a psychoeducational project adaptable to any system.

Adolescents' mental health in India

India is home to the largest number of adolescents in the world, comprising about a fifth of its population. According to the National Mental Health Survey of India, the prevalence of psychiatric disorders amongst adolescents is around 7.3% (Murthy, 2007). However, mental health difficulties remain one of the most neglected issues among adolescents in India, resulting in

DOI: 10.4324/9781003265610-8

increasing mortality and morbidity due to mental disorders at an alarming rate (Sivagurunathan et al., 2015).

Alongside the common issues rampant during this period of change, Indian adolescents face an abject lack of access to and availability of health care services. This situation extends to a lack of accurate information, proper guidance, and skills, as well as insufficient healthcare delivery systems and services, all of which are major barriers to adolescent mental health (Sivagurunathan et al., 2015).

According to World Health Organisation's (WHO) guidelines, one of the core principles of the Child and Adolescent Mental Health policy in India should be that the environment within and outside their residence and school be 'friendly' for optimum development (Hossain and Purohit, 2019) which, we suggest, includes taking an intersectional and psychosocial approach to mental health. However, given the country's vast diversity, this is challenging. Therefore, mental health workers aiming to practice with this population must be well-versed in the nuances of adolescent issues related to culture, family structures, financial background, language, and caste systems.

Another layer of difficulty in approaching this work is the social attitude formed due to the lack of information and infrastructure around mental health. In 2018, a study yielded a few important insights about the lack of mental health literacy in adolescent girls in India. It stated that in being unable to identify and label the problems as psychological or psychiatric conditions, sources of help for mental health problems become 'friends and parents, which begets inadequate knowledge about mental health services and treatments' (Saraf et al., 2018. p. 437). Adding to this is an allocentric culture that encourages adolescents to keep their issues to themselves or share them only with family members, further perpetuating stigma and impeding access to adequate mental health resources. As a result, there is an acute lack of awareness of mental health problems in Indian adolescents, and individuals with difficulties constantly express fear, shame, and sadness (Gaiha et al., 2020). This systematic review paper highlights the need for integrating mental health education into mainstream education by building awareness and sensitising youth through culturally appropriate methods.

Drawing on personal experience, we are aware of the efforts made by family members to keep their kin with mental health issues quiet. While these practices seem to be changing very slowly, the lack of psychoeducation has meant shame and malaise remain rampant. Through the National Health Mission in 2014, the government of India introduced school-based short programmes to improve adolescents' overall health. However, its inadequacy is manifested when addressing the mental health epidemic in the adolescent population (Hossain and Purohit, 2019).

Another need for intervention has emerged following the 'Right to Education (RTE) Act' (2009), which states that 'every child has a right to full-time elementary education of satisfactory and equitable quality in a formal school' This web site is referenced fully in the reference list. An abbreviated reference, for example: (Department of School and Literacy, 2009) might be more appropriate here within the text. This means that children from lower economic backgrounds are attending private schools. Nevertheless, the RTE Act does not provide due process for integrating them. Introducing such diversity without a supportive structure has left room for inequity. The resulting inequality vis-a-vis identity politics in classrooms has increased peer bullying (Malik and Mehta, 2016). The disparity between the rich and the poor has always played a huge role in inequalities in education in India, with most opportunities cushioned in the urban cities. On the other hand, children from rural areas and socially disadvantaged groups such as Scheduled Castes (SC), Scheduled Tribes, and Other Backward Classes (OBC) do not receive an equal number of opportunities in the educational system to succeed or realise their abilities, despite numerous governmental programmes aimed at reducing the gap between various socioeconomic categories (Bana, 2019).

The most current and prevalent mental health work in schools targets 'problematic' children. Therefore, counselling in schools is also viewed as a punitive rather than supportive measure. The lack of information also permeates the referral system and the counselling space, which is used to 'discipline' students. In contrast, the systemic issues that emerge in the classroom are not given enough attention unless they disrupt the class order. However, we believe the issue lies in inadequate measures for resolving underlying, fundamental, and pervasive issues. As Langs (1998) affirms, the framework within which the therapeutic context is set informs the practice itself as 'all the conditions of the context affect the status and operations of all the elements and the entities within the confines of the framework' (p. 3, 2019). This describes how the working alliance of the client – therapist dyad is affected by the cultural and political context, timeline, education systems, and what is considered acceptable social behaviour impacting both the client and the therapist.

The ensuing anonymised case vignettes exemplifies the many incidents that led the authors to develop Project Reflect.

CASE VIGNETTE 1 Psychoeducation and Morality

Anshuma: How are you feeling?
Chandan: I don't know. How does a person usually know how they are feeling?
Anshuma: Sometimes, our body can reveal how we are feeling. But sometimes it doesn't because we aren't feeling safe.
Chandan: Safe? What does that mean?

Chandan ran away from home when he was 14 years old. Growing up in a community of sex workers, he did not have the privilege of being child-like for very long. Finally, fed up with experiences of being beaten, bullied, and feeling that neither home or school was a safe environment, Chandan decided to risk venturing out into the world himself. 'How much more unsafe can it be out there?' he asked the friend who helped him plan his escape. However, within two weeks, he returned.

When the school nurse examined him, he had several unexplained scratches and bruises. He could not recount many parts of his experience. Unable to give the authorities any details of where he had been or what had happened, Chandan would only cry inconsolably anytime someone asked him where he had been. To date, no one knows these details.

Unfortunately, this case was not unusual. Chandran's school was part of a government initiative located on the outskirts of Delhi, in north India. It was specifically set up for the children of migrant workers, sex workers, and other poverty-stricken individuals and families who had built a slum community in this area. At first, the government tried to give them housing elsewhere, but they refused to move because they remained tied to their work, which was only possible at the fringes of urban society. While the government gave them aid and support systems such as schools, electricity, and healthcare options, the community remained rife with violence, drug-related issues, and crime. The authorities either looked the other way or blamed them for 'choosing' this life. A study on home-based sex workers and their children in India has shown them to be a 'highly vulnerable' population due to their poverty and exposure to high-risk sex and sexual violence. Safe spaces or care services from the public sector also remain inaccessible due to the illegality of their work in India (Hennink and Cunningham, 2011).

Children like Chandran were sent to school at the insistence of the social workers, albeit irregularly. For most parents, the school was considered valuable only as a place to safely remove the child from the home environment for the day. Conversely, schooling was seen by the authorities as an opportunity to teach the children the morals and values that their parents had not. The value systems of these two spaces were vastly different, and the children were expected to negotiate the gap. Instead, it led to confusion and feelings of alienation from both spaces. Violence and strife were the norms at home, while the school propounded sermons and prayer verses insisting on peace and non-violence written in big red letters all over the walls. Morning and evening prayers aside, the children also had to attend compulsory moral science classes and received frequent reprimands and detentions for their problematic behaviour.

At this time, Chandan was in class 8. As the son of one of the sex workers from the slum community, he was considered to be at the bottom of the social hierarchy and would often get bullied. He did not have access to his own space at home since his one-room 'kaccha' home (temporary structure) was also his mother's workspace, and he would often spend entire days and portions of the night out with other children or in the homes of neighbours. At school, he was quiet. In his few interactions with Anshuma, in her role as a part-time school counsellor and Drama and Movement Therapist, he would only state that both the home and the school made him feel like he was 'Nalayak' (not good enough).

Running away was a common occurrence amongst the school's students. However, Chandan's injuries, which included broken ribs, a concussion and suspected sexual assault, alarmed the school authorities. They decided to investigate the events, and Anshuma was also consulted to understand the necessary next steps as part of the measures undertaken. She proposed individual work and trauma-informed intervention for Chandan to establish a dynamic process that could include legal options, for example, alternative housing, if and when required. Alongside this individual intervention, she suggested a group process space where the students could express their feelings about the event. She also asked the school leadership, staff, and administrators to consider meeting the students to understand how to support them further. However, this latter proposal was deemed 'unnecessary'. The individual sessions were given the go-ahead, but instead of a group process space, a collection of students (including Chandan) considered to be 'difficult' or 'most likely at risk for being runways' were gathered, and Anshuma was asked to 'fix the problem'.

She understood that what was being called 'difficult' or even 'delinquent', was perhaps just confusion expressing itself through violence or escape. Given the lack of an enabling environment for age-appropriate social or emotional skill-building, the students were punished for 'acting out' because the overworked staff could not find time or space or had the skills to offer psychoeducational input. No one could focus on the larger, underlying issues in this volatile environment. Anshuma had to navigate the ethical dilemma of complying with the school authorities yet remaining true to the ethics of process-oriented, client-centred arts therapies.

CASE VIGNETTE 2 ***Psychoeducation and Privilege***

'I haven't read the Harry Potter books Abi, why don't you come out of the toilet and explain it?' Preetha said. Abi came out of the school toilet holding a blade in her hand, as she had self-harmed, again. She had been in therapy with Preetha for three years and had co-created safety measures, but it did not help her this time due to the intensity of her experience.

Initially, Abi arrived as a 'self-referral', saying she wanted to talk about her dynamics with her friends and use the space for self-exploration, as she struggled with extreme anxiety and recurrent panic attacks. She came from an affluent family who were always forthcoming when discussing Abi's struggles. Abi proactively engaged in therapy and was open to using creative arts therapies and exploring aspects of the body and gentle movement to regulate her emotions. She would bring in interesting metaphors, and her self-awareness and general outlook on mental health were quite expansive.

After Abi was coaxed out and given the necessary medical attention, the task was to talk to the class who had witnessed the entire incident. In this private school, they had a holistic vision of supporting children's overall well-being. The conjunction of management, staff, parents, and the children were quite strong, so they could always communicate and refer the child for mental health support. Though the school's major population falls into the upper-middle-class category, with the Right To Education (RTE) Act (2009, the school had a required percentage of students categorised under full scholarship from the lower-income group. Access to mental health support was for everyone.

As the predominant feelings of the class who had witnessed the incident were sadness, anger, confusion, guilt, helplessness, and fear, a whole class psychological intervention was designed to help the class process what they had witnessed, address mental health, focus on self-harm, and process these feelings using the arts. Since the probability of self-harm increases when children hear or witness others' self-harm (Fisher et al., 2012), it became crucial to check in on a few students individually and bring it back to the entire class to reflect on relevant mental health issues and topics. Using Arts Therapies helped create aesthetic distance in exploring safety, boundaries, empathy, and mental health.

The school's administration realised the need to compile a safety document focusing on self-harm. Though the Rashtriya Kishor Swasthya Karyakram (National Adolescent Health Programme) in 2014 under the Ministry of Health and Family Welfare had launched a programme ensuring holistic development of the adolescent population, the specifics of safety when addressing issues of mental health and self-harm had been overlooked. However, without much reference material and limited access to supervision, Preetha had to negotiate with the school, parents, peers, and students to make a culturally relevant self-harm protocol document. This solitary endeavour made it even more crucial for her to proactively seek collaborations from like-minded professionals in the field in India.

Though both authors worked in different economic, geographical, cultural systems, they realised the need for customisable psychoeducational projects. Project Reflect was the first of such endeavours.

The mental health of adolescents in India and the birth of Project Reflect

Many schools and institutions in India that did not earlier implement culturally relevant practices and ethical guidelines now give time and space to trained Mental Health First-Aid Professionals to develop interventions and best practices. However, we have observed that the norm in educational institutions for adolescents in India is that the authorities cannot specify a function for MHPs. As a result, these professionals sometimes become part of the disciplinary system or are used as substitute teachers due to the paucity of opportunity and lack of role clarity.

According to the Mental Health Atlas report by WHO (2017), there are 1.93 mental health workers for every 10,0000 of the general population of India, a situation which puts a tremendous strain on the Indian healthcare system, which in turn is unable to address the prevention of mental health issues (Singh, 2020). In addition, the scarcity of MHPs and the lack of a supportive infrastructure means these professionals have had to create community-based mental health programmes with a psychosocial approach. The reality is that there is inequality of access which means that while an urban Indian may have access to the 1.93 mental health workers, an individual from a rural part of the country does not. Barriers to implementation were identified as travel distance to receive care, limited knowledge about mental health, high level of stigma related to mental health issues, and poor mobile network signals and connectivity in the villages. Furthermore, a lack of familiarity with and access to mobile phones, especially among women, constitutes an obstacle to accessing health-related messages as part of the intervention (Tewari et al., 2021).

A research study in South Africa reveals a similar paucity of public sector mental health resources. It shows that participants of a psychoeducational mental health and well-being programme unanimously agreed to the importance of such a programme in their schools. Staff and school counsellors felt that the programme supported the behavioural and mental health issues of children whose families do not have the means to help their children with such services (Coetzee et al., 2021). Similarly, classroom-based psychoeducational programmes have contributed towards psychosocial and emotional development (Fazel et al., 2009). As arts therapies are non-threatening, have a playful approach, and normalise emotional expression, they enhance resilience, coping, self-esteem, and social behaviours that improve emotional and behaviour problems (Beauregard, 2014; Quinlan et al., 2016). One important feature of Project Reflect is that all children are positively engaged to promote inclusivity instead of addressing only children labelled 'difficult'.

Considering this, Project Reflect was started primarily as a classroom-based psychoeducational programme. Nevertheless, individual work or small group therapy formats felt more culturally relevant as we worked on the ground. We also realised how important it was to involve all the stakeholders in the adolescents' development (parents, teachers, students, and other staff). Therefore, alongside forming a research-based programme for the students, we also work with parents and teachers so that the programme can see long-term success. Studies show that school counselling programmes need evidence-based practices and policies, which can be achieved with more training and competence-building initiatives for school counsellors and teachers, which would in turn, improve their services (Vaishnavi and Kumar, 2018).

Given India's diversity of cultural paradigms, each context required a different approach. Therefore, the project had to be versatile, personal, and accessible. The choice of arts was for their expressive possibilities and also because Arts Therapies share a commitment to using physical and emotional expression as a therapeutic technique, harnessing creative energy for healing of the mind body and spirit, and belief in the power of creative imagination to navigate through difficult problems and conflicts (McNiff, 2004).

Project Reflect was conceived to bring the therapeutic and reflective aspects of the arts into classrooms through a programme designed to engage emotional intelligence and encourage empathy, inclusivity, and sensitivity in young minds. The aim was to develop a culture of emotional well-being within schools by engaging with all the stakeholders, to understand the needs to be addressed and devise a psychoeducational programme that could be delivered in the classroom. The result was an approach based on the principles of the arts therapies (Art Therapy, Dance Therapy, Drama Therapy, and Music Therapy) which combines these modalities with psychological and psychotherapeutic principles. The programme was then designed in progressive segments carefully adapted to the needs of the environment.

Theoretical underpinnings of Project Reflect

Although our respective education as Creative Arts Therapists differed, we shared ethical positions and the theoretical framework through which we understood the adolescents' problems. We both work from a psychodynamic lens, viewing mental health difficulties from a developmental, attachment-based, and trauma-informed approach. Being culturally sensitive and rooted in experience, we based Project Reflect on flexible theoretical paradigms that allowed movement and agency according to the particular needs of the setting. Thus, it constitutes a customisable programme that works within the system rather than outside of it. However, this does not mean that all the system's stakeholders are on board, and the workshops and training programmes aim to instil a way of thinking about mental health rather than prescribing it.

We found Maslow's (1987) hierarchy of human needs relevant to our work. Maslow conceived of human needs as a pyramid, ranging from 'physiological' at the base, ascending through 'safety', 'belonging and love', 'social needs', and 'esteem', to 'self-actualisation' and 'transcendence' (Crandall et al., 2020). In order to arrive at the next stage, the preceding one should have been satisfied. By organising our plans around the client's needs, we placed value on the urgency of intervention during the needs analysis. For instance, we included Mental Health First Aid (2017) as a part of our training so that students in distress could first be attended to, while the self-exploratory sessions came afterwards. Of course, not all students or schools opt for higher-order needs, so we specifically address other issues such as bullying. While doing so, we pay special attention to why the issue arose in this specific situation and the needs of this cultural context.

Thus, while psychoeducation is a model that encompasses some didactic elements, it also requires the practitioner to hold space for emotional and psychological aspects that get challenged or arise during the process. The structure that we proposed had a strong base in the arts therapies, including Chace's approach of structuring sessions in Dance Movement Psychotherapy (cited in Sandel, 1993); additionally, being observant of the body and movement using Laban movement analysis (North, 1990) was helpful to understand non-verbal cues. We also drew upon trauma-informed expressive arts therapy (Field, 2016) in response to a presented need. Furthermore, an integrated psychodynamic and humanistic framework, alongside Erik Erikson's psychosocial stages of development (1968), informed our facilitation of group work that addressed issues young people faced in schools and other environments.

Yalom's principles of group therapy (2008) have informed how we facilitate interpersonal learning within the group to make it even more context-specific and less dependent on the facilitator. For example, in Yalom's therapeutic principles, interpersonal learning amongst group members is a key therapeutic factor, as is the 'recapitulation of the family unit', which addresses interpersonal conflict and reflects familial and attachment-related conflict (Bowlby, 1984). In addition, giving space for individual work and allowing the students to engage in more personalised models of therapeutic drama, such as psychodrama (Moreno and Fox, 1987) and Developmental Transformations (Johnson, 2009), felt important and enabled empathy and insight, which sparked important psychoeducation topics as well as more contextually relevant group work.

Whilst the holding environment (Winnicott, 1953) allows expression, dialectical discussions, and processing through verbal and arts-based modalities, the overarching Project Reflect framework serves as a container for our trained counsellors and teachers (Bion, 2013). As their engagement with the students is continuous, we support them with tools that they can build upon and sustain as arts-based support for the students. When all of this goes hand in hand with psychoeducation around emotional regulation, adapting to physical changes in adolescence and to psychosexual developments, and dealing with anxiety, the student receives a well-rounded and holistic experience of personalised mental health care.

Erikson (1978) stressed that spontaneous, improvised play begins in the body. This experimental aspect of play transformed into symbolic acts helps develop relationships and social impulses (Piaget, 1998). Bringing play into the classrooms through the therapeutic impact of art forms, we also needed this model to be adaptable. Therefore, we decided that the ethos of Project Reflect will be strongly based on a need-based, flexible programme that school counsellors and class teachers on the ground could deliver. The framework would accommodate the 'here and now' of issues faced whilst providing a loose structure that could allow mental health education to be available in response to students' needs. The loose structure was also mindfully introduced to enhance the facilitator's innate ability to be creative and spontaneous and adapt to situations that might develop during the session. One such situation arose when a co-ed school reached out, saying there was a clear lack of engagement of their class 11 students (age 16) during class time. On observation and from in-depth discussions with the teachers, it was evident that the students were struggling with transitioning to college, anxiety around academic performance, and interpersonal challenges with their peers, which impacted their performance in learning and classroom presence. According to Erikson's developmental stage theory (1968), this is the stage referred to as 'identity versus role confusion' and an emphasis on adolescents forming their own identities as a result of their peer relationships (Rageliené, 2016).

Considering this, we planned whole class interventions addressing themes around mental health, transitions, performance pressure, emotional regulation, and interpersonal dynamics. We also addressed themes emerging from these topics, such as the upcoming end of school life, separations from friends, and worries about new beginnings. Again, we played the role of consultants. Arts Therapies approaches played a huge role in helping design sessions that the school counsellor and class teacher co-facilitated for the students in class. We noticed that though class interventions were planned, it was largely through the playfulness of the arts that children found it easier to engage, as processing their worries through the arts allowed them to verbalise their concerns rather than enact them in destructive behaviours and actions. As imitative behaviours play a vital role in group therapy formats (Yalom, 2008), the class started to model new acceptable behaviours from their peers and facilitators. Through supervision, we brought to the fore their challenging relational issues that helped the whole class move from old dysfunctional patterns to more empathetic and supportive ones.

Constant supervision with the on-ground staff and building a dynamic plan helped both the teacher and the counsellor to put certain strategies in place for emotional regulation. Though Project Reflect started as a short-term intervention programme, in some schools, it gradually became part of an expanding class curriculum. The project intended to embed mental health care's core values into the school system. However, once the school counsellors and teachers built this rapport and method of connecting with their students, they continued to evolve beyond our 'intervention' into a deep and resonant state of empathy. This evolution is apparent because even beyond the project, they continue to build tools such as feeling wheels, games, and nuanced and complex expressive arts activities that allow their expression and engagement to continue. As a result, we are now only consulted if they face a step requiring supervision.

When the pandemic hit in March 2020, India had a full lockdown, with all schools closing and reopening as online schools. This measure impacted unprivileged children, as they could not afford electronic devices or internet use. When onsite teaching slowly resumed after a year, the learning gap between underprivileged children benefiting from the Right to Education Act (2009) and more affluent children became even more prominent. The pandemic highlighted adolescent mental health, as quarantine made meeting friends and attending school impossible. As a result, there has been a surge in children's symptoms of stress, anxiety, and depression due to excessive worry, feelings of helplessness, loneliness, and a sense of collective unhappiness (Gore et al., 2021). The governments of different Indian states recognised this and suggested that schools deliver short psychoeducational programmes. This situation made Project Reflect more accessible for adolescents who otherwise disengage with mental health topics, as we support school counsellors in designing courses relevant to this particular group.

Adapting to the context and building a secure frame for creative arts therapies

In a country and a context that felt 'unsupportive', Project Reflect provided an itinerant service and laid the building blocks of a support system. Navigating complex systems of culture and systemic issues was a humbling process, and it became clear that this project, or any other endeavour, needed to be collaborative. Also, the country's sheer diversity and vast geography required all interventions to be adaptive and independent of specific staff. A spirit of collaboration, cooperation, and collective passion for seeing the field grow led us to establish The Arts Therapists Co-Lab (TATC), which supports arts-based, psychoeducational, and therapeutically oriented mental health ventures in India. So far, we have collaborated with established institutions and offered master classes to MHPs, teachers, artists, and others working with clinical and subclinical populations.

Privileges and opportunities

In our quest for mental well-being in children and adolescents in India, we have found ourselves amid systemic, seismic changes and have become part of the change. Nevertheless, we must pause to reflect and recognise our privilege to affect that change and have a voice. We are aware of our positions as educated, upper-caste, English-speaking, upper-middle-class women who could use our identities to express our minds. This reminder is important so that we do not perpetuate any discrimination but rather acknowledge our favourable position.

On returning to India as qualified practitioners, neither of us had envisioned that setting up our practice meant having to engage with establishing the field of work in the country. Most of us who have traversed the same path found no employment waiting upon our return, the very lack of available positions also constituted an opportunity. The scope of uncharted work in India meant that Project Reflect could access and collaborate across the country and its cultures to reach children and adolescents. The work ahead is both daunting and exciting as the field of Arts Therapies in India is in its adolescence. In conclusion, we hope to have initiated and piloted the beginnings of what could then grow into a field of practice that supports and sustains children and adolescents from all strata of Indian society. Project Reflect will stay committed to ethical client care, which the children and adolescents in India deserve.

References

Bana, A. (2019). *Socially Disadvantaged Groups and Poverty in India.* [Online] Law Corner. Available at: https://lawcorner.in/socially-disadvantaged-groups-and-poverty-in-india/

Beauregard, C. (2014). Effects of classroom-based creative expression programmes on children's well-being. *The Arts in Psychotherapy*, 41(3), pp. 269–277.

Bion, W. R. (2013). Attacks on linking. *The Psychoanalytic Quarterly*, 82(2), pp. 285–300.

Bowlby, J. (1984). *Attachment and loss* (2nd ed). Harmondsworth: Penguin.

Coetzee, B. J., Gericke, H., Human, S., Stallard, P., and Loades, M. (2021). What should a universal school-based psychoeducational programme support psychological well-being amongst children and young people in South Africa focus on, and how should it be delivered? A multi-stakeholder perspective. *School Mental Health*, 14, pp. 189–200. 10.1007/s12310-021-09465-3

Crandall, A. A., Powell, E. A., Bradford, G. C., Magnusson, B. M., Hanson, C. L., Barnes, M. D., Novilla, M. L. B., and Bean, R. A. (2020). Maslow's hierarchy of needs as a framework for understanding adolescent depressive symptoms over time. *Journal of Child and Family Studies*, 29(2), pp. 273–281.

Department of School and Literacy, The Right of Children to Free and Compulsory Education (RTE) Act. (2009). Available at: https://mhrd.gov.in/rte

Erikson, E. H. (1968). *Identity, youth, and crisis.* New York: W. W. Norton.

Erikson, E. H. (1978). *Toys and reasons: Stages in the ritualization of experience.* London: Boyars.

Fazel, M., Doll, H., and Stein, A. (2009). A school-based mental health intervention for refugee children: An exploratory study. *Clinical Child Psychology and Psychiatry*, 14(2), pp. 297–309.

Field, M. (2016). Empowering students in the trauma-informed classroom through expressive arts therapy. *Education*, 22(2), pp. 55–71.

Fisher, H. L., Moffitt, T. E., Houts, R. M., Belsky, D. W., Arseneault, L., and Caspi, A. (2012). Bullying victimisation and risk of self harm in early adolescence: Longitudinal cohort study. *BMJ*, 344(Apr 26 2), pp. e2683–e2683.

Gaiha, S. M., Taylor Salisbury, T., Koschorke, M., Raman, U., and Petticrew, M. (2020). Stigma associated with mental health problems among young people in India: A systematic review of magnitude, manifestations and recommendations. *BMC Psychiatry*, 20(1), pp. 538–538.

Gore, M., Swain, A., and Saraf, A. (2021). Has the COVID 19 pandemic exacerbated Indias mental health issues: A narrative review. *Annals of Medical and Health Sciences Research*, 11, pp. 114–118.

Hennink, M. M., and Cunningham, S. A. (2011). Health of home-based sex workers and their children in rural Andhra pradesh, India. *Asian Population Studies*, 7(2), pp. 157–173.

Hossain, M., and Purohit, N. (2019). Improving child and adolescent mental health in India: Status, services, policies, and way forward. *Indian Journal of Psychiatry*, 61(4), pp. 415–419.

Johnson, D. R. (2009). Developmental transformations: Towards the body as presence. *Current Approaches in Drama Therapy*, 2, pp. 65–88.

Langs, R. (1998). *Ground rules in psychotherapy and counselling*. Routledge.

Mahajan, P., Rajendran, P., Sunderamurthy, B., Keshavan, S., and Bazroy, J. (2019). Analyzing Indian mental health systems: Reflecting, learning, and working towards a better future. *Journal of Current Research in Scientific Medicine*, 5(1), p. 4.

Malik, A., and Mehta, M. (2016). Bullying among adolescents in an Indian school. *Psychological Studies*, 61(3), pp. 220–232.

Maslow, A. H. (1987). *Motivation and personality* (3rd ed). New York: Harper & Row.

McNiff, S. (2004). *Art heals: How creativity cures the soul*. Boston: Shambhala.

MHFA, Mental Health First Aid India (2017), (Online: Training Courses), Available at: https://www.mhfaindia.com/

Moreno, J. L., and Fox, J. (1987). *The essential Moreno: Writings on psychodrama, group method and sponteneity*. New York: Springer Publishing Company.

North, M. (1990). From personality assessment to dance education and therapy. *The Educational Forum*, 54(1), pp. 65–70.

Piaget, J. (1998). *Language and thought of the child: Selected works* (Vol. 5, 4th ed.). Taylor & Francis Group, Routledge.

Quinlan, R., Schweitzer, R. D., Khawaja, N., and Griffin, J. (2016). Evaluation of a school-based creative arts therapy program for adolescents from refugee backgrounds. *The Arts in Psychotherapy*, 47, pp. 72–78.

Rageliené, T. (2016). Links of adolescents identity development and relationship with peers: A systematic literature review. *Journal of the Canadian Academy of Child and Adolescent Psychiatry*, 25(2), pp. 97–105.

Sandel, S. L. (1993). Imagery in dance movement therapy groups: A developmental approach. In Marian Chace, Susan L. Sandel, and Sharon Chaiklin (Eds), *Foundation of Dance/Movement Therapy: The Life and Work of Marian Chace*. Amer Dance Therapy Association; First Edition, pp. 112–119.

www.nhp.gov.in. (2014). *Rashtriya Kishor Swasthya Karyakram (RKSK)/National Health Portal Of India*. [Online] Available at: https://www.nhp.gov.in/rashtriya-kishor-swasthya-karyakram-rksk_pg.

Saraf, G., Chandra, P. S., Desai, G., and Rao, G. N. (2018). What adolescent girls know about mental health: Findings from a mental health literacy survey from an urban slum setting in India. *Indian Journal of Psychological Medicine*, 40(5), pp. 433–439.

Singh, U. A. (2020). *Disentangling India's Mental Health Distress: Does India Have the Resources to Control the Impending Mental Health Crisis?* [Online] Research Matters. Available at: https://researchmatters.in/news/disentangling-india%E2%80%99s-mental-health-distress-does-india-have-resources-control-impending-mental

Sivagurunathan, C., Umadevi, R., Rama, R., and Gopalakrishnan, S. (2015). Adolescent health: Present status and its related programmes in India. Are we in the right direction? *Journal of Clinical and Diagnostic Research*, 9(3), pp. LE01–LE06.

Srinivasa Murthy, R. (2007). Mental health programme in the 11th five year plan. *Indian Journal of Medical Research*, 125(6), pp. 707–711.

Tewari, A., Kallakuri, S., Devarapalli, S., Peiris, D., Patel, A., and Maulik, P. K. (2021). SMART mental health project: Process evaluation to understand the barriers and facilitators for implementation of multifaceted intervention in rural India. *International Journal Mental Health Systems*, 15(1), p. 15. 10.1186/s13033-021-00438-2. PMID: 33557902; PMCID: PMC7871593.

Vaishnavi, J., and Kumar, A. (2018). Parental involvement in school counseling services: Challenges and experience of counselor. *Psychological Studies*, 63(4), pp. 359–364.

WHO. (2017). Mental health ATLAS 2017 member state profile. Available at: https://www.who.int/mental_health/evidence/atlas/profiles-2017/IND.pdf?ua=1

Winnicott, D. W. (1953). Transitional objects and transitional phenomena; a study of the first not-me possession. *The International Journal of Psychoanalysis*, 34, pp. 89–97.

Yalom, I. D., and Leszcz, M. (2008). *Theory and practice of group psychotherapy, fifth edition* (5th ed). New York: Basic Books.

Chapter 8

A safe portal of exploration for children and young people

The comic panel

Malcy Duff

Introduction

It is necessary to offer accessible resources that can be applied in different settings that will connect with a younger population. The comic panel is one artistic format that encourages creativity and is open for individual interpretation that a large group of people can access. In this chapter, I will explore the comic panel as a safe space for children and young people to tell their stories and frame their narratives. I will discuss the comic panel as a transitional tool and its connections to children's and young people's experiences. I will also consider the comic panel as one of the multiple physical and non-physical frames in an art therapy context that links well with psychoanalytic theories and finish the chapter with some suggestions for approaches using comic panels in a therapeutic environment (Figure 8.1).

The comic strip has been used in different contexts as an art form with huge potential in the therapeutic space. Examples include a CBT study which invited a group of children to use a comic strip to reduce anxiety around a mathematics test. Participants were encouraged to reflect on the causes of their stress, calmly dividing up time and overwhelming experiences into comic panels. The study found that the children could express chaotic experiences in a manageable way and observe associations, causes, and affect or change through comics, leading to an increased capacity to manage their emotions.

In Finland, existing characters were used for children to explore their inner feelings on justice and morals (Johansson and Hannula, 2014). The study questioned whether visual language would identify a stronger moral outlet than written stories. This non-directive use of character, although limited in this study, brings up important possibilities of how existing works can have identifiable qualities that can lead to personal expression.

Williams discusses whether comic book work can be cathartic or used as personal therapy (Williams, 2011). Through interviews with four cartoonists who have made autobiographical comic books around grief, trauma, and psychological illness, he asks what they feel the benefits of creating and

DOI: 10.4324/9781003265610-9

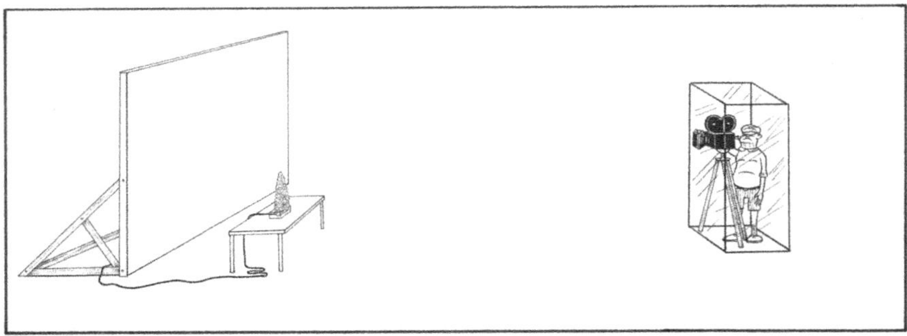

Figure 8.1

publishing these works have been. Narrative and memory within the comic book are discussed, and comics are found to be a useful communicative art form to share personal stories with others.

Gysin acknowledges this sequential art form's potential as a narrative therapy in that both approaches can 're-story' (Gysin, 2020). The author experiences the comic book as self-explorative through her journey using comics as art therapy and offers some possible applications for future clients in an art therapy context. Similarly, Carlton has chosen to use the comic book form as a medium of self-expression, appreciating that its format can offer containment, processing, and a reflective space (Carlton, 2018). Carlton also worked with clients, using the comic book form and its tools to give a space for the client to contain their work, a box for them to put their expressions. In this instance, Carlton used the computer programme 'Comic Life', which supplies ready-made panels, speech, and thought bubbles, meaning the tools are already there for the participant to fill. The study shows the comic strip's flexibility and strength as it offers choices and options through the participant's interpretation of the form. Shwed (2016) also argues that comic book storytelling can be a successful and versatile artistic approach in an art therapy context. She cites autobiographical works as examples of comics that communicate a person's lived experience. Using existing artworks in a session may allow participants to connect to the medium before attempting their own strips. Shwed suggests using pre-existing panels, speech, and thought balloons templates to encourage participants to create their comics.

The use of the comic panel as containing psychic skin, and the line of the panel creating a supportive structure for the contents, is explored through work with a client named Tanguy (Marotta et al., 2019). The comic strip's framing and framework are recognised as helpful in encouraging Tanguy, through his characters and story, to express his feelings. This article highlights that drawing a box on a page can lead to an explorative, creative process with links to psychoanalytic theory.

The comic panel

The comic panel is an integral part of a comic book. Cartoonists will use this format to structure a story and use it in the narrative flow capture events (Eisner, 2008), framing images and moments. It is the scaffolding the story leans on. The panel also captures duration within a single shot or still image (Smith, 2015). The size and shape of the panel may determine the amount of time passing within that frame. Often larger panels suggest a longer time span, and smaller panels depict shorter moments. The volume of panels on one page determines a sense of time and rhythm for the reader to respond to within the story's narrative.

The panel is a window into a story, and similar to a picture frame, it demarcates a specific section of a surface (Smith, 2015), the surface, in this case, could be the comic page. If we compare the comic panel to a window, we can consider it a window into specific states for the cartoonist and the reader. The cartoonist uses a comic panel as a window and interacts with it to discover a permanent image. They are opening the window to look out of it, breaking it, shattering the glass that divides the outside and inside, removing anything that prevents further exploration and entering it. The reader uses the window in more of a transitory way, like a passer-by peering in. The cartoonist and their story on a page is a house with windows, and the reader is a visiting neighbour.

The area around the panels is the space that the reader creates. If we consider the panels as windows of a house, the gutter literally becomes a gutter in the street surrounding those houses. The reader journeys past and around the windows (the panels), threading themselves through the in-between spaces (the gutter) and participating in the story by creating their personal interpretation of movement and sequence. The window page has been plotted to allow the reader portals into a story, the windows entry points, and gateways that the reader can easily access.

The reader's experience of the work is participatory. The creative process of making a comic can be split into three stages: the idea appearing, the creation of the comic, and then what the reader creates from reading the comic. The third stage, where the reader becomes involved, completes a creative cycle. The reader imagines what the story is and how it is being told by using the information they receive from the panels, and then use the gutter as a space for them to construct the narrative and develop its meaning. The reader has now become the creator. Their imagination now drives the story, and they fill the gutters with their images, the gaps between the panels now full of new possibilities.

There is the inner part of the panel inside the panel line and the outer part outside the panel line, but what of the panel line itself? What is the line? If we think about a cricket field, a boundary rope circles the pitch and delineates between in-play and out-of-play. The rope that is used as a boundary line is also a rope. The rope has substance and existence as a rope and is a functional element in the context for which it is used. It is a piece of rope with threads, knots, textures, and history.

The comic panel is similar in that the line clarifies the distinction between inner and outer, dividing space between cartoonist and reader, but should not be disregarded as purely functional. Like a rope on a cricket field, it also condenses substance and information into a single infinite line. Smith writes:

> 'Since the panel border is itself a drawn line, it becomes readily apparent that there is a kind of basic equality between the line that encloses the panel (providing a frame) and the depictive lines within that panel' (Smith, p. 231).

Within the panel line, we will find the person that creates what is within the panel.

The joined-up outline of a comic character divides space by saying this is part of a person and not part of the sky, and the line that does this is full of information. Skin textures, blemishes, hairs, and rag nails all exist within the outline of a character if we look closely enough. The cartoonist uses the same drawn line for the panel border, which may be the same drawn line used for drawing a character; therefore, the comic panel line is significantly connected to the information it wraps around. If inside the panel, we can see a person's inner experience, and outside the panel, we see the outer experience of the reader, the comic panel line settles in the middle between creator and reader. The line, therefore, describes part of the inner experience by selecting what we see and what the creator wishes to convey to us as readers, the reader's portal being the cartoonist's portal. The created space suggests walls, an environment, a boundary line, an encapsulation of experience, life, death, and even an afterlife, the line representing our duration, our lifespan. The panel line is the outline of a person (Figure 8.2).

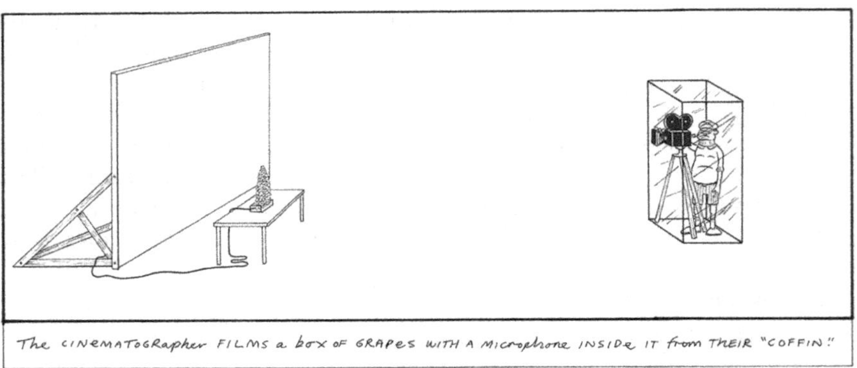

Figure 8.2 The cinematographer films a box of grapes with a microphone inside it from their 'coffin.'

The box and the panel

In early cinema, as silent films became talkies, the cinematographer suffered. Cinematographers who had previously wandered with their cameras, their lens floating through a story, were now required to stay close to where a microphone was placed. A microphone would be hidden in a piece of furniture or a flower vase, the effects of which are memorably satirised in the film Singing in the Rain (Nowell-Smith, 2017). The frame was now stuck.

The cinematographer's experience in the 1920s was made demoralising when they were placed in tomb-like soundproof boxes while on set, so the sound of their cameras would not be picked up by the sound recording equipment (Magid, 2019). Sound had destroyed the silence. This example of the early cinematographer in a box illustrates a space being imposed rather than created by the person that occupies the space, restricting creativity and diminishing collaboration. This box was a coffin, forcing the cinematographer into a new era while destroying what they once were.

Comic books and films use the frame as a portal into a story, with the reader or viewer experiencing the work via this frame. In film, storyboarding, finger frames, the lens of a camera, and a film strip through the lens of a projector are all processes that will involve framing an image until it lands at its final destination on a cinema screen. Comic books use the frame of the comic panel. This single direct frame is a way of plotting a story, organising a narrative onto the page and the portal the reader enters into the cartoonist's vision.

The framework involved in creating a physical box to one that is non-physical is very different. A physical box made for a person, by design, is restrictive. It is reflective of cages and jail cells, something that punishes and reduces free movement. It is also something we would find in a museum, a cabinet capturing an artefact to be distantly viewed now frozen in time. Creating a non-physical box can be a starting point that encourages creative freedom. This participatory box can be an entry point into another place, a space for exploration and imaginative journeys. The frame imposed around a person has very different implications for the structure built by the one occupying it. It highlights the many dangers of imposing a narrative onto other people's lives and placing a restrictive frame around creativity. The cinematographer in the box has been placed inside this space without choice. That frame now determines their existence and narrative. We must always ask, whose narrative is this and who creates this frame? How was this frame made, and what was the reason for it? The comic panel's framework and construction must be considered with this in mind (Figure 8.3).

Comic books and school settings

Comic book storytelling is an accessible art form that many children and young people are familiar with. The comic format continues to appear in many picture books for young children, with panels and speech bubbles used

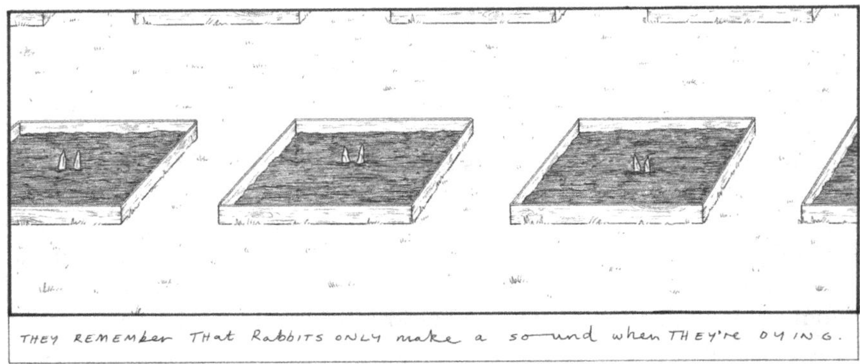

Figure 8.3 They remember that rabbits only make a sound when they're dying.

for narrative purposes. The 'Diary of a Wimpy Kid' series is one example of many popular books for pre-teens that use the comic book language in short strips running alongside prose and have been influenced by older newspaper strips such as Charles Schultz's 'Peanuts'. While graphic novels and other one-shot comic books continue to be hugely popular for adolescents, the comic book is finally getting the recognition in the U.K. it deserves as an important literary art form that can encourage reading and creating from a young age.

The comic book language is an effective communicative form to express individual experiences. The comic format has been applied in Carol Gray's Comic Book Conversations (Gray, 1994a) and perhaps most significantly in Social Stories (Gray, 2001b), which are now widely used as a standard communicative tool for children in mainstream and special schools across Scotland. PECS and Boardmaker in ASN schools in Scotland are examples of word and image combinations used for routine daily planners that acknowledge the importance of developing a visual language to increase verbal communication. Although these programmes apply generic templates, teachers and support workers will encourage children and young people to create picture symbols for their planners, individualising the templates through creative processes. This approach increases the scope of the form to represent actual lived experiences and reflect the individual accessing these tools.

The comic book bridges the visual and written narrative world in one concise form. Studies have shown that children on the autistic spectrum respond well to visual communication and comic book storytelling (Foss, 2016). The Homunculi Approach (Greig and MacKay, 2013), a CBT approach that encourages problem solving for participants by creating characters inspired by The Beano's Numskulls characters, is another visual communication tool currently used in ASN schools in Scotland. The participants are encouraged to develop their problem-solving strategies using characters

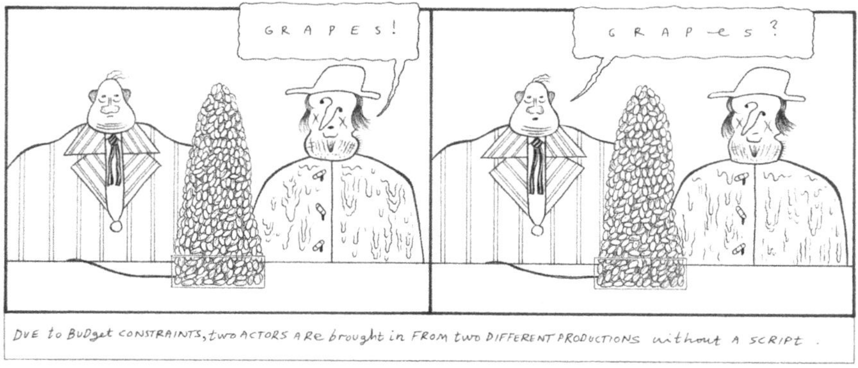

Figure 8.4 Due to budget constraints, two actors are brought in from two different productions without a script.

that reflect the representations in their minds and achieved through art making and comic strip templates that the participant uses to create a narrative.

The introduction of the Curriculum for Excellence in Scotland in 2010, a child-centred approach to learning, has seen an increase in the use of comic books in school settings. Several Scottish schools are now using comic books in their literacy curriculum. Cross-disciplinary work, particularly literature and artmaking combined, lends itself to using comic books as a learning tool. The combination of words and pictures that often make up a comic strip allows both artmaking and writing to thrive and support one another while exploring visual storytelling. Many learners may find writing and literacy very daunting, and comic making may be a way to increase their confidence by using a visual approach. A recent study used cut-out panels of pre-made comics in a school setting to develop learners' ability to tell a story (Wallner, 2018). A collaborative approach between learners and teachers was used, working together to put the comic panels in different orders to create new narratives from the existing work. This study showed that participants reading comics also become the producers of the work by focusing on the gutter on the comic page, as this is a place where individual interpretation and creativity can progress in different directions depending on the individual (Figure 8.4).

Comics and art therapy

In 1955 Donald Winnicott wrote to Charles Schultz to ask him permission to use his character Linus and his security blanket in Winnicott's writings on the transitional object. Winnicott saw something in the comic form that resonated with his work, and by referencing Schultz's hugely popular comic strip 'Peanuts', Winnicott acknowledged the use of the comic was an attempt to make a universal theory connect with a large group of people. He writes:

> 'A phenomenon that is universal ... cannot in fact, be outside the range of those whose concern is the magic of imaginative and creative living' (Winnicott, 2005, p. xvi).

Winnicott's referencing of Schultz's work is one example of the comic's range and ability to adapt to other practices while remaining accessible and unchanged in its original form. Winnicott focused on depicting childhood and the interaction of one character and a transitional object. He would also have seen the panel line enveloping Linus and his blanket, which makes his referencing possible and contains the possibility of further theoretical interpretation. It is interesting to consider what other comic strip elements connect with psychoanalytical theories underpinning art therapy practice. The use of comic book storytelling has been explored as a creative outlet in art therapy (Lucas-Falk, 2010; Hagert, 2017). The panel is the character that we often forget about, the inanimate scaffold that holds the comic world aloft, a line that creates a space where anything is possible. It is an open space, an opening that can be interpreted in different contexts and applied in many different settings.

Children and young people are going through constant transitions in their lives. The comic panel allows an ordering of change into a narrative sequence, and the organisational element of the panel may be a helpful tool for the child to use to structure transitions, especially when placed into a turbulent and overwhelming lived experience. The comic panel as a portal can reflect the transitional changes a child and young person will experience. The preparation for a transitional stage for the young person can involve a separation from a previous world into a new world (Van Gennep, 1960), and the comic panel can serve as a gateway into a new place, a liminal space for the child to investigate their experiences of change that mirrors the liminality of the therapeutic environment. Unlike a framed image, whereby the frame finishes the picture, the picture in a therapeutic context is not finished but part of a continuing story (Schaverien, 1989). The image in a framed comic panel is never finished and is part of an ongoing narrative. Although the comic panel and its contents are in a constant state of transition, the panel remains in a continuous and stable form. Stability and familiarity within a therapeutic environment may support a participant working through unstable experiences. In a physical environment, visible continuity and enduring symbols may give security to a person that may increase their ability to accept other possibilities (Lynch, 1982). The familiarity of working with a comic panel in each session can give continuity to the participant's work and may increase their confidence to explore transition within the therapeutic environment.

The therapeutic space is one set aside from daily life for an individual to allow themselves a meditative, silent, self-reflexive environment away from a material being, and the boundaries of a therapeutic session can prevent the process from becoming overwhelming for a participant and reduce any potential danger (Schaverien, 1999). The comic panel separates a space on the page by creating another frame in which the participant will subsequently work. The participant creates their own non-material space by creating this panel and, in doing so, creates their own therapeutic environment to work within, the panel itself reflective of a meta-therapeutic area, the page a 'meta-panel' (Eisner, 2008, p. 65). The comic panel uses a line to create a boundary around a participant's image and can be seen to reflect the boundaries of the therapeutic environment. There is a history of using boxes and frames in art therapy, and boxes are often used as physical containers for artwork (Farrell, 2001). Containment can be achieved through the therapy space, the art materials, and the artwork created in a session (Proulx, 2000; Stace 2011). The projection of an object into a container in a therapeutic environment can achieve containment (Bion, 1962), and the comic panel has been described as a 'container frame' (Eisner, 2008, p. 48). We can consider the comic panel to be another container applied in art therapy that can strengthen a sense of containment for the participant.

The panel bears witness to time passing and highlights the intricacies of an instance, inviting the cartoonist and reader to take time to increase their understanding of that moment. It can be presumed that anything continuous is divisible (Aristotle and Lawson-Tancred, 1998). The panel divides a lived experience into moments, allowing the constant to be broken, then stalled, paused for consideration, and reflected upon. The comic panel frames our stories and places them into digestible segments. The fragmentary nature of experience, where we perceive the whole but in parts, means the comic panel can give closure to overwhelming information (McCloud, 1994). Therapy exists in a particular frame and is separated for another purpose (Schaverien, 1999). By placing an image within a panel or drawing one around a specific image, we separate it from the whole. The closure this may bring for the participant in an art therapy context may make an overwhelming experience less daunting. The comic page brings the panels together to create the broken continuous of the comic book, the divided that stays whole. The comic page maps out a series of moments, presenting those parts together to create a united experience that can lead to reflection by asking questions about these moments and how they relate. We can ask ourselves what is happening in this panel, this moment, and then explore the before and after by adding more panels. How did we get to this place? Where will we go next?

The gap between the panels is a significant instigator of the comic's journey that encourages participation from the reader. These blank spaces on the comic page connect with the theories of analyst and author Marion Milner. Milner speaks of the 'framed gap' and the importance of recognising a frame in different contexts of human knowledge (Charles, 2012). These can delineate areas of perception from the inner and outer realities we experience. Milner describes the gap as the feeling one has when inside the creative process that is neither self nor other. The framed opening could be created by a blank sheet of paper (Pajaczkowska, 2008) and can increase the not knowing and absent-mindedness that leads to explorations in the subconscious. The reader of a comic page will comprehend and interpret the panels provided to them on the page, and in the sectioned gaps between, they will start to picture what is there. This white space becomes full of imagined images and possibilities created by the reader. The daydreaming of the reader that allows this to happen is as important to the story as the pictures the cartoonist has created; hence the reader and cartoonist exist together in a collaborative creative partnership. The reader swims on the surface of the page, diving into the spaces between panels and discovering what is in the in-between, submerging themselves in the gaps and emerging in the panels. As Milner (1972/2013) writes: 'one has to be willing to feel oneself becoming nothing to become something'.[1] Thus, to make the comic come alive, we must enter into nothing, the blank space where the reader can dream and create something.

The comic panel does not have to be read linearly. When we first look at a spread of panels on a comic page, we see many single instances all at once, inviting the participant to choose their own narrative. The cartoonist may create a linear story, but the reader can still read the work in a non-linear order. This possibility represents another important participatory aspect of comics where individual choice over interaction with the piece enriches the reading experience and opens the form up to non-traditional interpretation. Past and future exist on the same page, and the reader may choose in which order they experience this and determine the duration attended to the page. As the reader decides in what order they want to read the images, they also choose how much time to take over them. If we view time as a stream of pictures in flow (James, 2012), the comic page can represent how we experience time by using a collection of panels on a comic page fixed in a timeless space. This flexibility of the comic page, where the reader can jump back and forth in time, may be useful for a participant to reflect upon life events in sequence to consider how one event may relate to another.

Winnicott's theory of transitional phenomena has the potential to be explored further with the comic book language. External life and inner reality contribute to an interrelated space of experiencing (Winnicott, 1971). The testing of reality a child will work through to make distinctions between perception and apperception could also be applied to what we can do with a comic panel in a therapeutic environment. If we consider the inner reality to be interpreted as the inside of a panel and the external life of the gutter, the panel line could be perceived as the reality tester where we delineate between inner and outer reality and make decisions over what we consider to be separate from one another. When outlining a character, we also divide space into what we perceive it to be and something not to be. The line around the character's arm means we can differentiate it as an arm and not part of the tree in the background.

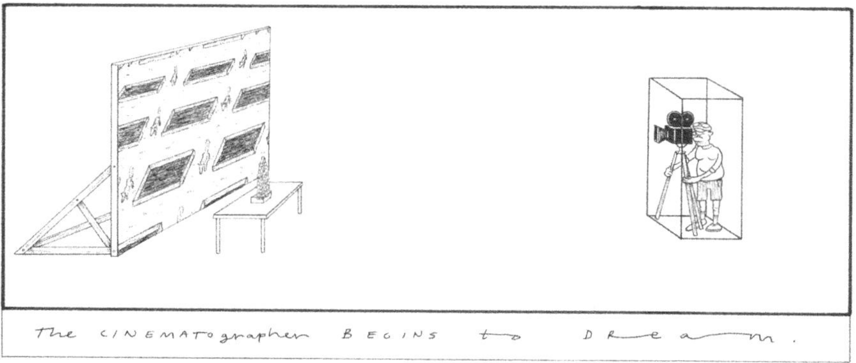

Figure 8.5 The cinematographer begins to dream.

Similarly, a child's reality testing within transitional phenomena allows them to decide what they perceive something to be, the inner me and the external, not me (Winnicott, 1971). The comic panel, therefore, can be seen as part of a transitional process that the child and young person can safely use to reality test, a non-physical transitional space that can be offered for play and exploration. Winnicott's referencing of Linus and his blanket can be viewed as a way of opening up the accessibility of the comic book to other theoretical interpretations that can deepen our understanding of working with children and young people in a therapeutic space (Figure 8.5).

The dog walking technique

In 2009 I began hosting workshops using a comic book approach I created called 'The Dog Walking Technique'. While designing this technique, I was particularly interested in the double-page spread in a printed comic book. When we open a double page spread, we are immediately hit with images from the past, present, and future within a story, which is unavoidable for even the most experienced comic reader.

Is there a way to create a unique panel in this spread that would give the reader a deep understanding of the story? This might be possible by introducing an abstracted panel to convey the essence of place and character in a single image related to all the other panels in the spread. I used the metaphor of a dog while meeting a dog walker and how we can get to know a person by getting to know their pet. I have been running this workshop for 12 years with children in schools across Scotland.

When offering this workshop in a time-limited space, I developed this technique with another thought in mind: how can a participant create a comic strip in a short time? The time constraints of a session can encourage you to think differently about how you create artwork. Working on a comic may take me three months from the initial idea to the finished book. This technique has helped me convey to a wide group of people the immediacy of the form and its possibilities, even within a limited time frame.

I begin the session with non-traditional experimental drawing techniques. These exercises, involving drawing while not looking at the page and drawing with your non-dominant hand, create a character. Once the character is visualised on paper, I work with the participants to develop their character, thinking about their attributes and what they would find in the world around them. I then ask them to create an inanimate object visually reminiscent of their character.

I introduce a double page spread full of empty comic panels at this stage. There are 11 panels, with a gap where the twelfth would be. This gap is the 'Dog Walking' panel. I encourage the participant to create a comic using the panels provided by asking them to combine the character and object as an inspiration for their strip, beginning by filling the space (The Dog Walking Panel) with the entity that reminds them of their character. The participant is now encouraged to think of a narrative combining the character and object. This idea of putting an object and character and putting them together to ask what will happen next is a simple starting point that can then be developed into a story.

The effect of presenting participants with panelled pages is interesting. Over these past 12 years, there has only been a rare occasion when these panels have remained empty. Participants use different approaches and mediums to fill the panels, including painting, drawing, collage, and writing, but whatever the method, images appear in the panels as if they have been waiting to be filled. This exercise and technique encourage creativity, and the introduction of the comic panel is integral to this happening.

As the sessions I facilitate in schools are often time-limited due to timetabling and other scheduling constraints, the work from the session may be continued after I have left the school. I will leave a page of panelled sheets for the school that can be easily photocopied and used in classes with their pupils after sessions. The comic panel can be easily duplicated and is accessible to teachers who may not have much experience in making artwork. They can be a structural starting point for more experimental expressive artmaking and literacy work (Figure 8.6).

Suggested approaches

The work that I have offered as a community cartoonist over the past 15 years informs my art therapy practice. Comic approaches have been used in some recent art therapy contexts (Hagert, 2017), and I hope that more work by therapists with a background in comic making and cartooning can

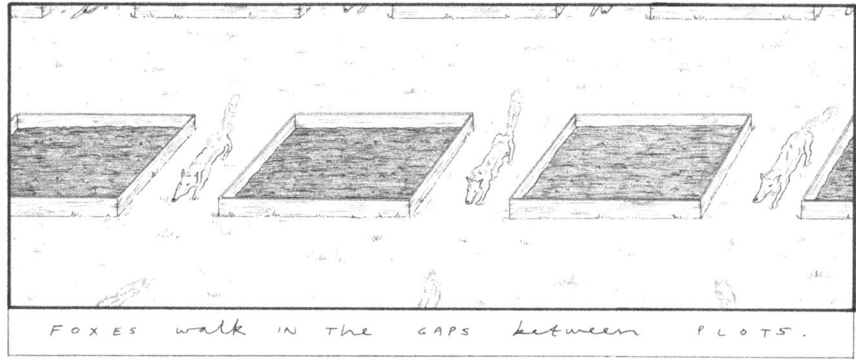

Figure 8.6 Foxes walk in the gaps between plots.

be offered. Applying this art form in therapeutic spaces has proven beneficial outcomes for participants. For example, for children and young people on the autistic spectrum, the comic book form can increase concentration and help with emotional difficulties (Greig and MacKay, 2013). However, there is huge potential for developing other approaches using comic book storytelling that are accessible for children and young people participating in art therapy and school and community settings and are also accessible to art therapists who may not have experience in making comic books. I offer some of these potential approaches below.

The panel is a mark on the page

The comic panel can be a supportive starting point for a person beginning to make artwork. The work may be the starting of a narrative or could be developed into other art making practices. In some art therapy sessions, I will offer a single comic panel at the beginning and invite the participant to use this as a space to work. The comic panel can be a way of focusing in, like a frame around a picture may separate it from the rest of the room (Schaverien, 1989); the comic panel may separate it from the page making the blank page less daunting. The comic panel becomes the first mark on the page that the participant can now add to and can be viewed as an encouragement to art making.

The panel as a 'check-in'

The panel can be used as a check-in at the start of a session, and this can be a way to engage in art making and focus on visual communication from the beginning by asking the participant to use colours that they feel represent their mood or using a descriptive image that captures their feelings on that day. The work can then further explore what is made within the panel, with the participant developing what they have made for the remaining session. The panel at the start of the session can be seen as a portal into the therapy session itself and a safe space to capture feelings and emotions.

The connecting panel

During the COVID-19 pandemic, I began sending panels through the post to participants to keep connected with the tactile elements of art making while working online and also keeping in touch with participants as some experienced intense isolation. Participants chose to use these panels to create stories or single images, potentially leading to larger projects that they could work into. I found it important to draw these panels by hand, making the panel unique and unlike any other, reflecting the importance of the participant and that I am keeping them and their individual therapeutic experience in mind.

The panel as optional art material

Careful consideration should be given to how the comic panel is introduced in a session. The panel shouldn't feel like an imposition on the participant but an invitation into a safe working space. I have attempted this by placing panelled comic sheets alongside blank sheets of paper when setting up an art therapy space, the comic panels being another option for the participant should they want to explore them. These pre-panelled comic pages will be offered as any other art materials in the room, an open invitation allowing the participant to decide whether or not to use them like they would for any other material. Participants interested in making comics and feeling more confident may want to create their panels. The therapist can support this and encourage the participant by supplying materials and advice about approaches and techniques.

The panel as a pictorial diary

The therapist offering a comic panel is an acknowledgement of the therapeutic frame for the participant, recognising its limitations and reflecting the length of therapy. In some therapeutic work, I will create a sheet of panels with the number of panels corresponding with the number of sessions the participant will be attending. We begin each session by encouraging the participant to make a piece of artwork within the panel to acknowledge the number of sessions we have left together to order the therapeutic intervention into an accessible artistic process that may be helpful for participants who feel overwhelmed by the length of therapy and help them prepare for the end of treatment. This Pictorial Diary of the therapeutic experience can be reflected upon between participant and therapist as therapy concludes and support a participant to acknowledge their progress and experience in the therapeutic frame.

The next panel

'Scientist / Potion / VCTM' was a comic strip I created in 2011. The strip centres around one frozen moment in time between three characters, the scientist, the potion and the VCTM. The strip's narrative is continued in panels under the large image with questions about that frozen moment, asking what is happening in the image and imagining possibilities. This strip's format also encourages working in a comic form by taking a single picture that is created in session and then asking the participant to make a comic strip about it. The participant may explore what is happening in that image and what happens next, with a comic strip flowing from the initial picture and leading to further exploratory work.

Conclusion

The comic panel is an accessible art form that encourages creativity and participation. Its functional line is also full of condensed information that can be applied in many settings, including the therapeutic environment. The panel is an opening, and its application in a space creates another space, a portal leading us further into imaginative territory. Its openness invites a participant's interpretation to be expressed, and its soft direction can encourage creative work. It contains elements of transition and closure that may be particularly helpful to the young person experiencing transitory states. The comic panel also reflects the therapeutic space, fits into a history of the uses of boxes in an art therapy context, and can connect with many psychoanalytic theories that underpin art therapy practice. At this time of a mental health crisis in our young population, we must continue to strive to find graphic formats that are open and available. The panel is waiting to be filled (Figure 8.7).

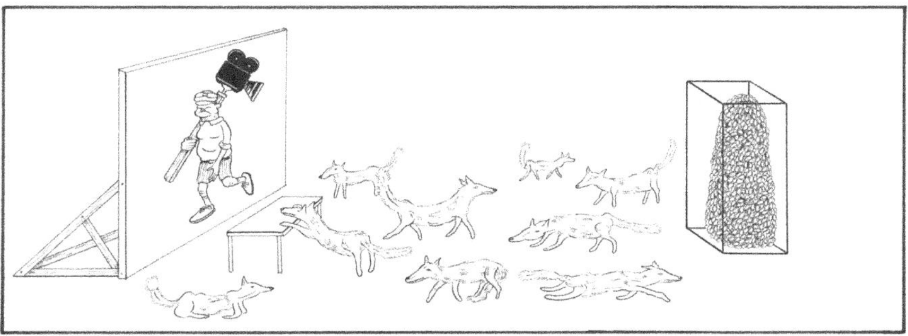

Figure 8.7

Note

1 'I found myself using the diagram with its empty space between the two lines as a way of reminding myself how emptiness, formlessness, must be the basis of new forms, almost perhaps that one has to be willing to feel oneself becoming nothing in order to become something.' (Milner, 2013, p. 180).

References

Aristotle and Lawson-Tancred, H. (1998). *Metaphysics*. London: Penguin Books.

Bion, W. (1962). *Learning from experience*. London: Karnac Books

Carlton, N. R. (2018). Illustrating stories: Using graphic novels in art therapy research and practice. In S. Imholz and J. Sachter (Eds), *Psychology's new design science and the reflective practitioner*. Rover Bend, NC: LibraLab Press. pp. 110–129.

Charles, M. (2012). Marion Milner: A life of one's own; an experiment in leisure; on not being able to paint; the hands of the living god: An account of a psychoanalytic treatment; eternity's sunrise: A way of keeping a diary. *The American Journal of Psychoanalysis*, 72(3), pp. 287–304. 10.1057/ajp.2012.15.

Eisner, W. (2008). *Comics and sequential art: Principles and practices from the legendary cartoonist*. New York: W.W. Norton.

Farell-Kirk, R. (2001). Secrets, symbols, synthesis and safety: The role of boxes in art therapy. *American Journal of Art Therapy*, 39(3), pp. 88–92.

Foss, C. (2016). Reading in pictures: Re-visioning autism and literature through the medium of manga. In C. Foss, J. W. Gray, and Z. Whalen (Eds), *Disability in comic books and graphic narratives*. Basingstoke, Hampshire: Palgrave Macmillan. pp. 95–110.

Greig, A. and MacKay, T. (2013). *The Homunculi approach to social and emotional wellbeing*. London and Philadelphia: Jessica Kingsley Publishers.

Gray, C. (2001b). *The new social story book*. Arlington: Future Horizons.

Gray, C. (1994a). *Comic strip conversations illustrated interactions that teach conversation skills to students with autism and related disorders*. Texas, US: Arlington Future Horizons.

Gysin, S. (2020). *Panel by panel: Changing personal narratives through the creation of sequential art and the graphic novel*. Quebec, Canada: Concordia University, Montreal.

Hagert, E. (2017). An exploration of art therapy process with a detainee diagnosed with schizophrenia in a correctional facility with reference to the use of the comic strip. In K. Killick (Ed), *Art therapy for psychosis*. New York: Routledge. pp. 181–202

Hinz, L. D. (2017). The ethics of art therapy: Promoting creativity as a force for positive change. *Art Therapy*, 34(3), pp. 142–145. 10.1080/07421656.2017.1343073.

James, W. (2012). *The principles of psychology. Vol. 1*. New York: Dover Publications.

Johansson, J. and Hannula, M. S. (2014). How do Finnish children express care and justice in comic strips and written narratives? *Journal of Moral Education*, 43(4), pp. 516–531. 10.1080/03057240.2014.900481.

Lucas-Falk, K. (2010). Comic books, connection and the artist's identity. In C. H. Moon (Ed), *Materials and media in art therapy: Critical understandings of diverse artistic vocabularies*. New York: Routledge. pp. 231–256.

Lynch, K. (1982). *What time is this place?* Cambridge: MIT Press.

Magid, N. P. (2019). Image makers: Documenting Hollywood's early masters of light. American Cinematographer, Feature, November 6, 2019. https://theasc.com/articles/documenting-hollywoods-early-masters-of-light
Marotta, J., Bonnet, C., and Gimenez, G. (2019). Tanguy et le cadre de la case. *Psychothérapies*, 39(2), pp. 93–100. 10.3917/psys.192.0093.
McCloud, S. (1993). *Understanding comics: The invisible art*. New York: Harper Collins Publishers.
McCloud, S. (1994). *Understanding comics: The invisible art*, (reprint edition, April 27, 1994). New York: William Morrow Paperbacks.
Milner, M. (2013). Winnicott: Overlapping circles and the two-way journey, a paper presented a memorial meeting for D.W. Winnicott, given to the British Psychoanalytical Society in 1972. In: J. Abram (Ed), *Donald Winnicott today, the new library of psychoanalysis*. London and New York: Routledge. pp. 246–252.
Nowell-Smith, G. (2017). *The history of cinema: A very short introduction*. Oxford: Oxford University Press.
Pajaczkowska, C. (2008). On humming: Reflections on Marion Milner's contribution to psychoanalysis. In L. Caldwell (Ed), *Winnicott and the psychoanalytic tradition*. London: Karnac Books. pp. 33–48.
Proulx, L. (2000). Container, contained, containment. *Canadian Art Therapy Association Journal*, 14(1), pp. 3–6. 10.1080/08322473.2000.11432243.
Schaverein, J. (1989). The picture within the frame. In A. Gilroy and T. Dalley (Ed), *Pictures at an exhibition*. London: Routledge. pp. 147–155.
Schaverien, J. (1999). *The revealing image: Analytical art psychotherapy in theory and practice*. London; Philadelphia: Jessica Kingsley Publishers.
Shwed, A. (2016). Crisis averted in infinite lives: Utilising comics as clinical art therapy. *Intima: A Journal of Narrative Medicine*. Available at: www.theintima.org
Smith, G. M. (2015). Comics in the intersecting histories of the window, the frame, and the panel. In D. Stein and J. Thon (Eds), *Comic strips to graphics novels' contributions to the theory and history of graphic narrative*. Berlin, Boston: De Gruyter. pp. 219–238.
Stace, S. M. (2011). Confusion and containment: Art therapy with an adolescent hospitalised with paediatric neuropsychiatric systemic lupus erythematosus. *International Journal of Art Therapy*, 16(1), pp. 52–57. 10.1080/17454832.2011.570271.
Van Gennep, A. (1960). *The rites of passage*. London: Routledge & Kegan Paul.
Wallner, L. (2018). Gutter talk: Co-constructing narratives using comics in the classroom. *Scandinavian Journal of Educational Research*, 63(6), pp. 819–838. 10.1080/00313831.2018.1452290.
Williams, I. (2011). Autography as auto-therapy: Psychic pain and the graphic memoir. *Journal of Medical Humanities*, [online] 32(4), pp. 353–366. 10.1007/s10912-011-9158-0.
Winnicott, D. W. (2005)(2nd Edition). *Playing and reality*. London and New York: Routledge.

Chapter 9

'The sun keeps on shining'

An experience of dramatherapy with ASD pre-adolescents

Rita Pirovano

Introduction

Before graduating in dramatherapy, I worked as a Neuro-Psychomotor therapist for more than 11 years at Villa Santa Maria, a Child and Adolescent Neuropsychiatric Institute near Como, Italy. The Institute cares for over two hundred residents and outpatients suffering from different conditions, such as neurodevelopmental delays or disorders, psychopathologies, and congenital and acquired cerebropathies. These are very complex pathologies; however, in most cases, knowing the causes and recognising the symptoms is sufficient to set up a clear and straightforward treatment and rehabilitation plan. The same cannot be said of Autism Spectrum Disorders, which currently affect about 60% of our guests.

It is not easy to identify the most appropriate approach in the case of ASD children, both because of the complexity of the condition itself and the huge variety of individual symptoms. Over the years, I have repeatedly experienced the frustration of feeling ineffective or inadequate in seeking advice from colleagues and supervisors; thus, I have changed my way of working and being with autistic children several times. However, the experience provided me with a greater willingness to listen and allowed me to open up to more questions and accept that it is not always possible to find an answer. I started studying Dramatherapy with the aim of finding a new perspective that would complement my knowledge and tools.

Dramatherapy with ASD children

Autism spectrum disorder (ASD) is a developmental disability characterised by persistent impairments in social interaction and the presence of restricted, repetitive patterns of behaviours, interests, or activities (APA, 2013). ASD affects 1 in 54, with four males diagnosed for each female in North America (Christensen et al., 2012), while the prevalence in Italy is 1 in 87 children aged 7–9 years (Narzisi et al., 2018).

DOI: 10.4324/9781003265610-10

To date, there is no universal standard treatment for ASD, but there are different approaches. The main ones are the psychodynamic-psychoanalytic approach (Bettelheim, 1967), the behavioural approach, which includes the Applied Behaviour Analysis (ABA) (Lovaas et al., 1978) and the evolutionary, naturalistic behavioural interventions.

The last ones, conceived around the 1980s (Schreibman, 2015), include many techniques, the most renowned being the Teacch program (Schopler and Mesibov, 1984).

In recent years, the interest in dramatherapy applied to groups of ASD children and young people has been growing. Tytherleigh and Karkou (2009) reported positive outcomes in their case study on relationship building with young people on the autistic spectrum in a special school. Participants benefited from role play, projective techniques, and interactions within the group to explore one-to-one and whole-group relationships.

Greene (2012) showed that engaging with dramatherapy for ten weeks significantly improved the ability of children to keep calm when facing difficult situations, and parents reported an improvement in their child's ability to show empathy towards them. Similar results were reported by Godfrey and Haythorne (2013), who provided an evaluation of post-therapy outcomes through the use of audio-recorded semi-structured interviews; there was no negative feedback, and improvement was noted in main areas: increased confidence and self-esteem, improved sense of self, increased opportunities to develop creativity and imaginative thinking, improved cooperation and turn taking, greater social and communication skills, improved skills to work effectively alone and with others. Dooman (2017) employed the Behavioural Assessment of Social Communication of Young Children (BASCYC) scale to measure the outcomes of interventions that she undertook with two groups of children aged 5–7 years in primary school settings. Specifically looking at responsiveness, she reports that results from the BASCYC scale provided quantifiable evidence that dramatherapy had a positive impact on the early social behaviour of ASD children.

In this chapter, I will describe a dramatherapy workshop devised for a group of ASD children/pre-adolescents, focusing on specific objectives and showing its effectiveness as a tool to help the clients to recover some key abilities.

Structure of the workshop

The dramatherapy workshop, consisting of 23 sessions with a group of five subjects with autism of different severity, outpatients of the Institute, was accompanied by an experimental study. The study evaluates the outcome of the workshop through the combined use of specific scales for autism and the assessment of dramatic abilities.

In particular, we analysed the effects of dramatherapy on the following areas:

1 Difficulties in storytelling
2 Difficulties in the recognition, expression, management, and representation/verbalisation of emotions
3 Poor tolerance for frustration
4 Poor self-awareness
5 Rigidity of thought and action related to limits in imaginative thinking and creativity

Evaluation tools

In order to evaluate the effects of Dramatherapy treatment, we used quantitative and qualitative tools.

Quantitative tools

Observation grid on individual dramatic skills with the addition of some items related to specific objectives for the specific context.

This grid was formulated in 2010 by the Italian dramatherapist Salvo Pitruzzella. It allows one to assess the skills acquired by a subject in the dramatic process. It classifies dramatic skills into three areas related to some fundamental elements of drama: Role, Expression, and Interaction.

Specific dramatic features are assessed for each of the three areas:

- Role skills include concentration in playing a role, the distance from the role, and the role's coherence and complexity.
- Expression skills include the personal use of space, facial expression, body movement and vocal/verbal expression.
- Interaction skills include involvement (entering the game), communication (listening and being listened to), exchange (accepting the contributions of the other and responding adequately), and cooperation (working together).

The intrinsic qualities of each area are safety and flexibility: the closer you move towards a balanced set of skills, the more confident you become in expressing yourself and flexible in your interactions (Pitruzzella, 2014).

For the purpose of evaluating additional specific skills related to the objectives of the project, we added an Emotional area, which considers the expression and mentalization of emotions, the tolerance to frustration and the variability of mood.

The grid is filled in by the therapist at the end of each session and discussed with the co-therapist.

Psychlops questionnaire

Initially created at the King's College in London and furtherly reworked by Roundabout Dramatherapy, Psychlops is a questionnaire designed as an outcome measure for mental health treatments, assessing the person's well-being by taking into account the subjects' ability to recognise, express, and mentalise their emotions, and their level of self-awareness.

Three versions of the questionnaire had been issued: for children (age 7–13), adolescents (age 13–16), and adults. The children's version is colourful and appealing; many items are facilitated by the use of emoticons. It allows children to express themselves creatively in answering certain questions.

The questionnaire consists of three domains (Problems, Functioning, and Welfare) and only four questions are scored. The other questions provide useful qualitative information but are not used for the calculation.

The maximum score for each question is 4 in the children's version (0 to 4) and 5 in the adolescent version (0 to 5), while the total score range is 0 to 12 in the first version and 0 to 20 in the second. The higher the score, the more the person is suffering.

The total pre-therapy score is compared to subsequent scores (during therapy and post-therapy). The difference between total pre-therapy and post-therapy scores represents the 'change score'.

CARS scale

The CARS scale (Childhood Autism Rating Scale) is a widely used tool developed by German-American Psychologist Eric Schopler to identify autism in children at an early stage and distinguish it from other developmental impairments (Schopler et al., 1986). It consists of 15 items concerning the main behavioural areas: relationships with others, imitation, emotional response, use of the body, use of objects, adaptation to changes, visual response, auditory response, taste-smell and use and response to touch (using and responding), fear and anxiety verbal communication, non-verbal communication, level of activity, level, and consistency of intellectual response, overall impression. To each of them, a variable score from 1 to 4 is assigned; the sum of all the scores gives a total value, which states the level of autism from light to severe.

In our project, the CARS scale has allowed the monitoring of emotional skills, tolerance to frustration, imitative skills, and flexibility.

The CARS, developed and tested on more than 1,500 cases over a period of 15 years, also has the advantage of being simply taught to operators with little experience in autism.

Qualitative tools

6PSM (six-pieces story making)

This tool, in several ways, responds to the need for a rapid evaluation of coping strategies, with the aim of helping the therapist/operator to set up a relationship based on understanding the user's 'inner language' (Lahad, 1992). Lahad suggests the following simple procedure:

> 'We are going to tell a story without words. What I mean is that you scribble or draw the story in any way you wish, following my instructions (questions). There is no need to worry about how nice the drawing is or if it can be understood, you can always explain it. (Note—the story can be told in words).
>
> a Divide the page into six spaces in any way you want (but do not cut it).
> b Think of a main character—hero or heroine of any story; imaginary, legendary, film, show, or simply make one up. Think about where this character lives as this will be the first picture.
> c The second picture will be the mission or task of that character. In every story or legend, the main character has a task to fulfil. What is your hero/heroine's mission?
> d Third picture. Who or what can help the main character, if at all?
> e Fourth picture. Who or what obstacle stands in the way of his/her carrying out the mission/task?
> f Fifth picture. How will he/she cope with this obstacle?
> g Sixth picture. Then what happened? Does it end or continue?
>
> Those are the six parts of the story. Now, with lines, shapes, symbols or drawings, compose your story. When you have finished, you can explain it to me (there are no time limits) (Lahad, 1992: 156–7).'

The focus is on the coping modes that emerge in the story. The most frequent are usually the most developed by the subjects in their everyday coping with stress.

In our project, through the use of 6-PSM, we monitored the ability of the child to invent a story or remember and tell/represent it; it is also useful to evaluate imaginative skills, creativity, coherence, cause-effect relationships, and sequentiality. It has been proposed by the therapist before and after the whole workshop in an individual setting within a safe and neutral space.

Clock of emotions

This is a clock created by the therapist using a plastic card cut into a circle, on which six different facial expressions have been glued in circular order in emoticon mode (very happy, happy, neither happy nor sad, sad, very sad, angry); at the centre is placed an arrow with a clasp that allows to move it pointing it towards the faces.

It is used both for monitoring the children's well-being and promoting their ability to recognise their own emotions and those of others and to represent and communicate their state of mind.

Repeating this activity regularly allows children to increase their mastery of the tool itself, which they learn to use with ease and spontaneity.

Each child, at the beginning and end of every single workshop session, is asked to point out the expression that best represents the emotional state in the here and now. The child, after having indicated the expression, can simulate it with his own face and name it by changing his own tone of voice; he is also asked why he feels so. The expressions indicated by the individual children are pinned on a card created specifically for each meeting in order to better highlight the responses of the individual at the beginning and end of the single session.

The group

The members of the group were initially six, aged between 9 and 16 years, with a primary diagnosis of Infantile Autism, according to DSM V criteria and validated through ADOS-2, associated with a mild/medium intellectual disability. We will call them by the fictitious names of Tommy, Abdelah, Giuseppe, Nicolò, Daniele, and Felice. Some of them had already attended a theatre workshop I had led for two years, where I had gradually introduced dramatherapy techniques. After seven meetings, the multidisciplinary team agreed on removing a member (Tommy) from the group since different needs emerged, to be further investigated through individual therapy.

All five boys use verbal language, which in the case of three of them (Nicolò, Daniele, Giuseppe) is communicative, while in the other two cases (Abdelah but above all Felice), it is mostly characterised by echolalia. All have already done group activities in the centre and show potential in the relational sphere, although significant nuclei of isolation remain, varying from case to case. A difficulty they have in common, although to different degrees, is the ability to recognise and express emotions. This difficulty correlates with a poor tolerance to frustration, which in some cases can manifest itself in the form of anxiety, with crying and moaning, and sometimes with provocative and aggressive behaviours. There is also a rigidity of thought and action that often results in repetitiveness, generating further frustration.

The sessions

The sessions have been led by me with the support of a colleague Neuro-Psychomotor therapist, in a large, cosy, and bright room of the gym inside the Institute. At each session, the boys are accompanied to the room, where they sit on the benches and take off their shoes.

Each session is organised according to the three-fold structure that also characterises the entire process of dramatherapy, including the stages named Foundation, Creation, and Sharing.

In the foundation stage, people experiment with the basic languages of drama; in the creation stage, they are free to devise scenes out of their imagination, playing roles and inventing stories, while the final stage of sharing is dedicated to de-role-ing, exiting from dramatic reality, and to a common recapitulation of the process.

In the foundation stage of our workshop, a coloured parachute was placed on the ground in the centre of the room at each session, and, one at a time, the boys were invited to sit on a wedge of different colours, forming a circle. I had explained to them how this figure is very important because, in the circle, everyone sees everyone, without anyone in particular being the centre of attention. The circle is an 'emotionally safe place' where people learn to listen to each other and express their emotions (Mosley, 1998).

Once seated, the clock of emotions is passed hand to hand, and each boy is given time to tell how he feels.

Subsequently, they greet each other according to a playful modality suggested by the therapist (for example, by passing a magic stick and saying their name, varying the volume and tone of the voice).

They are then helped to recall the experience of the previous session in order to improve their awareness of the process as a whole.

At the centre of the parachute, there is a 'magic pot', a sort of blue cauldron containing material which can be useful to set up the dramatic reality.

The creation stage is introduced by a story as told by the therapist, which serves as a narrative framework. The story sees the initial protagonist a little witch, personified by the co-therapist, who owns the 'magic pot' with which anyone can be turned into a hero. The story is told during the first four sessions in order to foster the creation of the heroic characters. Gradually, each boy is helped to invent his hero, identifying his mission and discovering his resources and helpers, making him face difficulty and deciding the conclusion of the story. A detail is added at each session to characterise the hero, for example, his distinctive object, costume, name, motto, and mission/task. Then, with the support of the therapist and the collaboration of the group, each of them can experiment with his own mission and eventually reflect on what he has discovered and learnt in the process.

In consideration of the traits of rigidity of the children of the difficulties in managing frustration and solving problems, we gradually propose variations, transformations, obstacles, limits, and negations. However, children are free to accept or reject a proposal and are supported to express both pleasant emotions and unpleasant emotions or difficulties. In the construction of roles, we suggest exercises and games to promote their expressive skills in terms of the use of the body, voice, gaze, and facial expressions. Observation of the other and imitative skills are stimulated through pretence play and 'as if'.

In the sharing stage, de-roling activities are carried out, the clock of emotions is proposed again, and we greet each other by standing up and throwing the parachute in the air; finally, we return to sit on the benches to put our shoes back on.

By the end of the workshop, a little performance is prepared to be shown to an audience of people they know, both peers and adults.

In the final sessions, a greeting party is organised for the various heroes, in which they can see the video of the final performance and comment on it.

The case of Daniele

I would like to discuss the results of the workshop and my feelings during the dramatherapy process by telling you about the case of Daniele, a teenage boy who has been attending the Day Centre of Villa Santa Maria for about ten years. He presented childhood autism and mild mental retardation as a clinical diagnoses.

From a motor point of view, Daniele is slow, clumsy, and rigid; he can imitate only simple gestures. On a relational level, he is able to call by their name people he knows, seeking adults to satisfy his needs and desires; he shows likes and dislikes for peers. In his free time, he prefers to play alone with building bricks or to leaf through illustrated books. If stimulated by the adult, he is willing to participate in group games and activities. However, it is clear that Daniele does not have a 'theory of mind', meaning that he is not able to put himself in someone else's shoes.

At a cognitive level, Daniele is able to read, even if not very fluently, to copy and write simple texts under dictation, although he shows difficulties in attention. He has a low threshold of tolerance to frustrations: when at school he is scolded or corrected, he gets angry, sometimes cries or engages in mild aggressive attitudes: for example, he kicks the classmate in front of him or throws objects on the ground. In some moments of inactivity, verbal and motor stereotypies have been observed.

He has limited communicative intentionality: he expresses himself mainly using verbal language, based on simple sentences, with monotonous prosody. During the pretend play, Daniele proves to be able to modulate his gestural and facial mimicry (which is sometimes excessive) and to use different voices depending on the role played.

Results

The results are described below, divided by quantitative and qualitative tests, focusing in particular on Daniele.

Summary of quantitative tools results

From the analysis of the data collected through the **Dramatic Abilities Assessment Grid**, there is generally greater adequacy of individual dramatic skills or, in some cases, maintenance of the starting skills.

In particular, several aspects are greatly improved in Daniele: the ability to elaborate the role, the investment of space, the expressive skills through modulation of facial expressions, the involvement in interaction, the expression and mentalisation of emotions, and aspects related to flexibility in action and thought (Figure 9.1).

From the results of the administration of the **Psychlops Questionnaire**, it is clear that a greater level of well-being has been achieved for most of the children. In particular, Daniele was able to state that the concerns initially recorded did not bother him at all, which looks like a great improvement compared to what he had said at the beginning, that it was difficult for him to do anything because of his problems, saying he felt very well in the last week and much better than before the therapy (Figure 9.2).

Analysing the results of the **CARS scale**, we can notice that, in general, for all children attending the workshop, a decrease in the level of autistic symptoms is observed at the end (in particular, two subjects have passed from a medium grade level of autism to medium-mild, another maintained a severe level, a quarter from medium to mild and a fifth from severe to medium).

Daniele is more open to social relationships, imitative skills, emotional responses, and the use of his own body and objects (in terms of variability and creativity) slightly improved, while his ability to adapt to routine changes slightly worsened (the educator reports that the child bursts into tears when faced with a sudden change in routine); skills related to verbal and non-verbal communication, at the activity and intellectual level, are stable (Figure 9.3).

	Dramatic Abilities Assessment Grid											
	ROLE			EXPRESSION			INTERACTION			EMOTION		
NAME	B	M	E	B	M	E	B	M	E	B	M	E
Daniele	7	8	10	10	10	10	8	9	9	6	6	6
Felice	4	4	4	16	9	10	8	8	8	6	4	6
Giuseppe	4	5	7	5	8	8	8	8	10	6	5	7
Nicolò	12	8	10	7	8	9	9	9	11	7	6	9
Abdelah	4	4	4	16	16	12	13	12	12	9	8	6

Figure 9.1 Dramatic abilities assessment grid.

	Psychlops Questionnaire											
	Problem 1			Problem 2			Functioning			Wellbeing		
NAME	B	M	E	B	M	E	B	M	E			
Daniele	5	0	0	3	0	0	0	0	0	0	0	0
Felice	/	/	/	/	/	/	/	0	0	0	/	0
Giuseppe	5	5	0	5	0	0	5	5	0	0	0	0
Nicolò	5	3	2	5	1	3	5	3	2	5	3	2
Abdelah	2	3	4	/	/	/	4	0	4	0	2	0

Figure 9.2 The results of the psychlops questionnaire with the same five children.[1]

	CARS Scale	
NAME	Pre	Post
Daniele	37/60	33/60
Felice	57,5/60	47,5/60
Giuseppe	36,5/60	32,5/60
Nicolò	37/60	31,5/60
Abdelah	43/60	34/60

Figure 9.3 This grid shows the pre and post results of the CARS scale.

Summary of qualitative results

Emotions clock

By analysing the responses provided by each child at the beginning and end of each session, there is generally an improvement in their ability to recognise, express and justify their emotions, gradually becoming aware of themselves and, in some cases, of the others' mood.

Daniele uses the tool adequately, referring to his mood related to the present moment. During the course of the treatment, he has always stated that he was very happy both at the beginning and at the end of the session, generally explaining at the beginning of the session that the reason for his happiness depends on being there with his friends, or on an external event (an activity carried out at home with his family or that he will carry out, or an environmental condition or because it is his birthday) or by his own physical condition (for example he verbalises that he is very happy because a little beard is growing under his chin). Instead, he usually links the happiness at the end of the treatment to the activity just carried out, specifying which detail he appreciated most or what he learned (for example, how to overcome his mission). At the beginning of the final performance, he states that he is very happy for the start of the show and, in the end, he declared himself happy to have celebrated and greeted the superheroes.

6-PSM

Analysing the results of the 6-PSM, it is evident in general, a tendency to spontaneously take inspiration from the stories of the heroic characters constructed during the treatment, illustrating more or less coherent stories, sometimes limited to drawings and words, others times well-constructed, represented and narrated with care and creativity. The results of Daniele's 6-PSM are analysed below.

At the beginning of the treatment, Daniele's imaginative repertoire is restricted to a known heroic figure, or Superman. The mission, the resources and the conclusion appear to be coherent, but the child is unable to hypothesise possible obstacles and, therefore, ways of overcoming them. Neither social nor cognitive, nor affective resources emerge. At the end of the treatment, it is observed that Daniele, after having listened, experienced and dramatised the story conceived and represented in the performance, shows that he is able to represent it graphically in sequential terms and narrate it easily by marking the different passages with linearity and coherence. Some details are included in the representation, for example, the vibration of the bell that rings and the still clapper of the bell that fails to have an effective sound; happiness is represented on the hero's face, sadness in the face of the frustration of not being able to reach the goal and the final joy, shared with other people, in being able to carry out one's mission. Behind the guide of the story constructed and represented with the adult and the companions, Daniele is, therefore, more easily able to exploit his own cognitive and emotional-relational resources, including the others' social resources, in solving the problem.

Conclusions

I was swinging inside a tunnel looking at the lights projected on its walls by the sound and light game of Winny the Pooh. I have been several times in that tunnel with Daniele, I well remember how that was one of the few ways to capture his attention and try to establish a relationship with him based on shared pleasure. Only gradually, over the years, through neuro-psychomotor treatments integrated with educational ones, I started to see more and more glimmers of light, up to proposing a drama-therapeutic activity to him.

'The sun keeps on shining' is the title of the final show and, I would add, of my therapeutic experience with Daniele and of the dramatherapy group.

I started the laboratory full of energy, radiant like a sun, eager to put into practice theoretical studies, games, and activities and test the evaluation tools identified in the previous months. Unfortunately, darkness soon appeared: the important emotional-relational and behavioural difficulties of a member of the group, Tommy, destabilised the group. I thought several times about the primary objectives of the workshop, one of which was to promote a state of greater well-being, and at that moment, Tommy was not feeling well in the group and his companions could have been affected by his inner discomfort. The choice therefore fell on the decision, taken in agreement with a multidisciplinary team, to have Tommy follow a different path. And here, recognising and respecting my emotions, I was able to face the initial difficulty and go back to seeing the light.

I tried throughout the whole workshop to convey to the children the importance of trying not to get stuck in front of an obstacle but to recognise it, accept the possible help of others to face it and come out of it as heroes, perhaps a bit bruised, but proud to have tried to overcome it. We were able, both me and the boys, to work on our rigidities and blocks, struggling to tolerate certain frustrations, get help and bring a contribution of novelty. All in a playful way, having fun, perhaps not always understanding the request but letting oneself be guided by the charm of imitating others. With a smile, the desire to get involved and a gaze directed towards the light, I would therefore invite you to read and reflect on the message left by one of the boys on the last day:

> *'Dear hero, if life puts you to the test, always remember that ... the sun keeps on shining!'*

Note

1 Daniele, Giuseppe, and Nicolò filled out the Questionnaire in the version for adolescents, while Felice and Abdelah the version for children.

References

American Psychiatric Association. (2013). *Diagnostic and statistical manual of mental disorders* (5th ed). Arlington, VA: American Psychiatric Association.

Bettelheim, B. (1967). *The empty fortress. Infantile autism and the birth of self.* New York: Free Press.

Christensen, D. L., Baio, J., Braun, K. V., et al. (2012). Prevalence and characteristics of autism spectrum disorder among children aged 8 years — Autism and developmental disabilities monitoring network, 11 sites, United States, 2012. *MMWR Surveillance Summary*, 2016(65), pp. 1–23.

Dooman, R. (2017). Assessing the impact of dramatherapy on early social behaviour of children on the autistic spectrum. In D. Haythorne and A. Seymour (Eds), *Dramatherapy and autism* (pp. 137–155). London: Routledge.

Godfrey, E. and Haythorne, D. (2013). Benefits of dramatherapy for autism spectrum disorder: A qualitative analysis of feedback from parents and teachers of clients attending roundabout dramatherapy sessions in schools. *Dramatherapy*, 35(1), pp. 20–28.

Greene, J. (2012). An educational psychology service evaluation of a dramatherapy intervention for children with additional needs in a primary school. In L. Leigh et al. (Eds), *Dramatherapy with children, young people and schools: Enabling creativity, sociability, communication and learning* (pp. 195–205). London: Routledge.

Lahad, M. (1992). Story-making as an assessment method for coping with stress: Six-piece story-making and BASIC Ph. In S. Jennings (Ed), *Dramatherapy: theory and practise 2* (pp. 150–163). London: Routledge.

Lovaas, O. I., Young, D. B., and Newsom, C. B. (1978). Behavioral treatment of childhood psychosis. In B. Wolman, J. Egan, and A. Ross (Eds), *Handbook of treatment of mental disorders in childhood and adolescence* (pp. 385–420). Englewood Cliffs, NJ: Prentice-Hall.

Mosley, J. (1998). *Quality circle time*. Cambridge: LDA.

Narzisi, A., Posada, M., Barbieri, F., Chericoni, N., Ciuffolini, D., Pinzino, M., and Muratori, F. (2018). Prevalence of autism spectrum disorder in a large Italian catchment area: A school-based population study within the ASDEU project. *Epidemiology Psychiatric Sciences*, 29, pp. 1–10.

Pitruzzella, S. (2014). *Mettersi in scena*. Milano: FrancoAngeli.

Schopler, E., Reichler, R. J., and Rochen Renner, B. (1986). *The childhood autism rating scale (CARS) for diagnostic screening and classification of autism*. New York: Irvington.

Schopler, E., Mesibov, G. B., Shigley, R. H., and Bashford, A. (1984). Helping autistic children through their parents: The TEACCH model. In E. Schopler and G. B. Mesibov (Eds), *The effects of autism on the family* (pp. 65–81). New York: Plenum.

Schreibman, L., Dawson, G., Stahmer, A. C., Landa, R., Rogers, S. J., McGee, G. G., Kasari, C., Ingersoll, B., Kaiser, A. P., Bruinsma, Y., McNerney, E., Wetherby, A., and Halladay, A. (2015). Naturalistic developmental behavioral interventions: Empirically validated treatments for autism spectrum disorder. *Journal of Autism and Developmental Disorders*, 45(8), pp. 2411–2428.

Tytherleigh, L. and Karkou, V. (2009). Dramatherapy, autism and relationship building; a case study. In V. Karkou (Ed), *Arts therapies in schools: research and practice* (pp. 197–216). London: Jessica Kingsley.

Chapter 10

Working with LGBTQIA+ Youth in Residential Settings

Diedré M. Blake

Introduction

This chapter explores furthering the discussion on the use of arts therapies with LGBTQIA+ (lesbian, gay, bisexual, transgender, queer/questioning, intersex, asexual/aromantic/agender, and those not specifically mentioned) youth. This exploration is undertaken through examining the research on LGBTQIA+ youth, including literature specific to arts therapies with this population, and my reflection on my experience as a trainee art therapist in the northeastern US from 2004 to 2006. Although I continued to work with this population after my training, I decided to focus on this specific period because it was the point when I knew the least about what to do. The circumstances for LGBTQIA+ youths and adults in the US and elsewhere have drastically changed over the past twenty years. Still, much needs to be done in and outside of arts therapies. In my work, five themes emerged that may be useful guideposts for fellow therapists.

Within the U.S. mental health care system, LGBTQIA+ youth remains a significantly underserved community (Green et al., 2020). Although lack of affordability and parental approval remain major barriers to receiving mental health care for LGBTQIA+ youth, there are also concerns about the importance of practitioners' multicultural competence in understanding their needs that I came to realise during my training as a graduate student from 2004 to 2006 and subsequent work as an individual and group expressive therapist (Green et al., 2020; Yarhouse et al., 2018). It is proposed that multicultural competency lies at the heart of how arts therapies professionals can find ways to better serve this community to give adequate care to diverse groups of people, especially youth (Wing Sue and Sue, 2008).

Creating space for LGBTQIA+ youth in residential settings to be themselves is vital. Although the focus of my graduate training was in art therapy, utilising a variety of creative arts modalities was significantly beneficial for clients because they were not limited to having only one mode through which they could express themselves. Using art, music, movement, writing, and film allowed clients to explore themselves, develop skills, and engage with each

DOI: 10.4324/9781003265610-11

other in new ways. The focus of this chapter, however, is not on practical tasks but on sharing how the current and past literature aligns itself with the following themes:

1 Social displacement
2 Challenges to finding community
3 Changing self-identification
4 Embracing new modes of self-expression
5 Bridging the multicultural gap.

I have placed particular emphasis on social displacement, challenges to finding community and bridging the multicultural gap to be at the core of commencing therapeutic work with LGBTQIA+ youth in residential settings. For the themes of changing self-identification and embracing new modes of self-expression, I have limited my discussion primarily to my observations and suggestions for working with this theme rather than an in-depth exploration. Therefore the tasks shared in this chapter are limited in their inclusivity and may need to be modified for differently abled clients.

I explore these identified themes sequentially with reference to some of the relevant literature and illustrate them with vignettes from my practice, followed by a description of a creative arts task. This use of the literature will help to retrospectively illuminate some of the issues I encountered in practice from a more current perspective.

A Little Background: An Entry Into Group Homes & Residential Programmes

During my graduate studies, I worked in two residential settings for adolescents, one was a group home exclusively for LGBTQIA+ youths, and the other was a mixed residential care programme. At that time, I was a trainee, learning about expressive therapies (also known as creative arts therapies and arts therapies). specifically art therapy. My background was solidly rooted in art and LGBTQIA+ activism rather than psychology. However, I believed in the healing power of art and wanted to find a way to help young people in and outside of the LGBTQIA+ community. As such, I was delighted that I could do so in the two aforementioned settings. As my experiences and thoughts cannot represent the entirety of any topic, I have punctuated my reflections with the inclusion of supplementary literature, which can provide further insight into each discussion point.

To the outside world, the group home would have appeared as any other large suburban home where several teenagers (ages 13 to 18) lived. The only differences would have been the 24-hour presence of staff members supervising all activities and the fact that the teenagers seemed to be unrelated. These teenagers went to school regularly, were taught vocational skills by staff members and also trained at local shops in the community. The ultimate goal for residents in the group home is to have a safe place to call home while preparing to become independent young adults. During my time at the group home, for those residents, the group home was a place where they could exist without judgement, explore their identities, and work through the various internal and external challenges they faced. Certainly, many of them did not want to be there. However, being there was often seen as a better alternative to being at home or being on the streets. I saw residents who were able to reunite with their families. I saw residents who were adopted by new families. I also saw residents who aged out of the group home and had to transition into adult services.

The residential care programme was part of a broader wrap-around services programme, working to improve the lives of children (ages 6 to 18) and their families. In this programme, there were residents and non-residents, children who stayed in the programme and children who remained at home but participated in programme activities and events. As a trainee, my work involved individual therapy, group therapy, and home visits. With this approach, the programme worked to provide comprehensive care such that residents and non-residents could experience living at home in a safer and more nurturing manner. As with the group home, the residents and non-residents were from diverse backgrounds and had diverse identities and challenges.

I saw many residents become non-residents and non-residents transition out of the programme. Arriving and leaving (and sometimes returning) could happen very quickly. In general, the average length of stay for the group home at the time I was based there was between 3 months to 6 months. For the programme, it was between two weeks to two months. Of course, there were outliers, residents who only remained for a day or two or residents who stayed for a year or more. What can be said for all of the youths I met is that they were all seeking someone that they could trust and some place where they could be safe, especially feel safe to express themselves.

Around the mid-1990s, Donna Addison (1996) and Rachel Brody (2013) published articles in Art Therapy on the use of art therapy with homosexual clients. In the early 2000s, literature on the use of art therapies with the LGBTQIA+ community was still quite limited (Pelton and Sherry, 2008). Moreover, the discussion on the need for evidence-based practices in arts therapies was still in its infancy (Gilroy, 2006). As such, my approach to working with LGBTQIA+ youth became a matter of trial and error–trying one modality and then another or even mixing, whether in individual or group therapy. Primarily, I used art, music, and writing in individual therapy. In group therapy, I added reading and watching films specifically related to LGBTQIA+ themes. Watching films related to coming out (accepting and sharing one's sexual and/or gender identity with others), in particular, appeared to help even the quietest of group members to discuss their experiences. For myself, it was through these individual and group therapy discussions that I began to identify what seem to be the core themes of LGBTQIA+ youths in residential settings: social displacement, challenges to finding community, changing self-identification, embracing new modes of self-expression, and bridging the multicultural gap.

Social Displacement

If I were to summarise the questions of many of the youths I met during (and after) my years as a trainee, the summary would be, "who am I, and where do I belong?" Perhaps for the LGBTQIA+ youths I met, I would tweak the summary to be, "who am I … if there is nowhere I belong?" Many LGBTQIA+ youth in the U.S. have experienced social displacement, whether literally or metaphorically (having a home and family but feeling isolated within those structures), leaving them without a sense of belonging but with a feeling of profound helplessness (Choi et al., 2015). It is estimated that, in a given 12-month period, approximately 1 in 30 youths, ages 13 to 17, experiences homelessness, i.e., unaccompanied by a caregiver (Morton et al., 2017). The estimates are worse for young adults ages 18 to 25, 1 in 10 of whom experience homelessness (Morton et al., 2017). LGBTQIA+ youths have a 120% risk of reporting homelessness due to conflict in the home as a result of their sexual identity or gender expression, which leads to either being forced out of their homes or running away from their homes (Choi et al., 2015). Furthermore, youths who identify as African American/Black, Latino(a)/Hispanic, or Native American are overrepresented, regardless of sexual orientation or gender identification (Choi et al., 2015; Morton et al., 2017; Youth.gov, n.d.).

The term *social displacement* is used within the fields of communication studies and sociology, respectively, as a hypothesis and perspective to describe the impact of disruption to the individual or collective sense of belonging (Hall et al., 2019; Smith, 2010). My use of the term *social displacement* is more simplistic, only requiring the consideration of the implication of the combined words: *social*, meaning "of or relating to people or society in general," and *displacement*, meaning "the situation in which people are forced to leave the place where they normally live" (Cambridge Dictionary, n.d.; Merriam-Webster, n.d.). Furthermore, I would contend that displacement can be applied to an emotional experience as well, rather than just a physical experience. The questions I asked at the beginning of the section may well capture the emotionality of the experience of the LGBTIA+ youths with whom I worked, who may have been feeling socially displaced, having a sense of groundlessness, a lack of belongingness, and a gnawing sense of anxiety about their identities.

Based on the data on homeless and unaccompanied youth, LGBTQIA+ youths are more likely to find themselves forcibly removed, whether directly or indirectly, from their accustomed social environments and have to find or create new communities. Certainly, considerable progress has been made in the acceptance and inclusion of sexual minorities in the U.S., and more members of the LGBTQIA+ community can count on support from both their families of origin and families of choice (Hull and Ortyl, 2019). However, the challenges that LGBTQIA+ youth face as a result of family rejection remain significant. For example, compared with non-LGBTQIA+ youths, LGBTQIA+ youths are at a higher risk of developing physical and mental health problems or struggling with issues such as substance abuse, depression, suicidality, and self-stigma (Katz-Wise et al., 2016). As such, providers, including arts therapies professionals, may find that addressing the experience of social displacement may become a part of their work with LGBTQIA+ youth. However, what could this look like in practice?

Residents in a Group Home and a Residential Programme

As a trainee, I had the opportunity to work with residents both as an individual and group therapist. Many of the young people living in the residential settings where I trained self-identified as LGBTQIA+ and had been placed there by the state department of children and family services. The residents in both settings came from low to middle socioeconomic backgrounds primarily and were racially diverse, although, in the group home, there were more youths of colour in comparison to the residential programme.

For the group home, the primary reason for placement was due to conflict in the home directly related to their sexual and/or gender identities. In fact, some of these young people had already been homeless by the time of their admission, others had been removed from their homes, while others still were voluntarily placed. In the residential programme, the youths were placed due to conflict within the home, not necessarily related to their sexual or gender identities. As such, the youths in the residential programme did not all identify as LGBTQIA+. In both settings, I met with residents once or twice per week, depending on the group and individual therapy scheduling.

Both in individual and group therapy, participants often spoke about the anxiety of the unknown and not knowing where to go. There was a sense that there was no home to return to and no new home where they could go. Some clients held a strong sense of ambivalence towards their families and their fellow residents. Moreover, there was a lack of trust in self and others, and anger about their circumstances. Opening up to others was difficult. I found that therapy sessions started from the aforementioned emotional states: ambivalence and anger. Thematically, however, I thought that the idea of not knowing both 1) home and 2) who they could trust could be explored through art therapy and may offer a path towards resolution.

In response, I proposed that residents explore the idea of creating a home within themselves through art. Not only did the residents explore creating a home within themselves, but also creating a home within their new setting. In addition, group work, using mandalas and collages, helped to create connections and improve social skills. Individual work involving self-portraits (current and future) also appeared to be useful for residents. Also, offering open studio hours, in which residents could choose for themselves what they wanted to do, reinforced that residents had a say in their lives and could exert control over some aspects of their lives. Certainly, the above activities described were and are not groundbreaking. At the time, however, I had unlocked something within the residents, who, through connecting with art and discussing their creations with each other, seemed to develop a better understanding of each other and themselves.

I would like to address my thoughts about myself as a therapist in training at that time. To be honest, as a trainee, I sometimes felt fearful of what would happen in the next individual or group therapy session. There were many thoughts that ran through my mind at the time. *Would there be only silence in an individual session? Would someone act out and start a fight in group therapy? Did I have enough tools to allow for exploration and expression? Was I good enough? Did I even belong here? Will they ever trust me?*

Through supervision and my own art process, I was able to address my feelings of fear, inadequacy, and frustration. I also learned a valuable lesson from my supervisor at the residential programme, who explained that it was my job to learn about each person, their background, their goals, and their needs before trying to work towards any solution. Although we spoke of "residents," the residents were not a monolith. I took that lesson to heart and worked towards being more open, acknowledging that I had not been looking at each person as an individual. Furthermore, I understood that I had to learn that one resident's feeling of social displacement was not the same as another resident's.

Challenges to Finding Community

I have mentioned that LGBTQIA+ youth of colour are overrepresented in the number of youth who report homelessness and accessing homelessness services (Green et al., 2020; Morton et al., 2017). This data corresponds with my observations of the youth residential settings in which I worked.

In these settings, the majority of clients identifying as LGBTQIA+ clients also self-identified as either African American/Black, Latino(a)/Hispanic, or biracial/multiracial. Some described themselves as having been previously homeless or having been repeatedly removed from their home and placed in foster care or other residential settings over a long period of time. For LGBTQIA+ youth not identifying as being members of a racial minority group, some described similar experiences, while others were experiencing being displaced for the first time. This information is merely anecdotal. However, it serves to underscore that the current data aligns with the circumstances I encountered between 2004 and 2006 and leads to the next theme that emerged in my work with these young people: finding community.

There are various ways in which the word *community* can be defined. For the purpose of this section, I would like to focus on five elements that were found to be important in making a community in an article on community collaboration and HIV vaccine trials by Macqueen et al. (2001). To understand and better foster community collaboration in HIV vaccine trials, Macqueen et al. conducted qualitative interviews with 113 participants to identify what community meant to them. Their findings resulted in identifying five key elements that make a community:

Key elements defining community (Macqueen et al., 2001)

1) locus, a sense of place, the physical space of community, e.g., a neighbourhood or a local recreational space 2) sharing: common interests and perspectives, having an understood value system, 3) joint action, a sense of cohesion and identity, unintentional and intentional working together as a community that creates cohesion, 4) social ties, the foundation for community, interpersonal connections, e.g., family of origin and family of choice, and 5) diversity: social complexities within communities, not specific to race or ethnicity, but focused on a broader scope of differing levels of interpersonal relationships as well as demographic differences.

MacQueen, K. M et al. (2001, p. 1931).

For all youth in residential settings, finding community, i.e., a sense of belonging to a specific community in which they can fully participate, can be challenging. For LGBTQIA+, however, the challenge can be especially demanding. Residential settings are, for the most part, transitional experiences. Young people have been placed there until a more permanent housing or foster care option can be found or the difficulties facing their families can be resolved. It is not typically intended for long-term care. However, there are many young people who remain within these settings until they effectively age out of the child welfare system and therefore must leave their residential setting and live independently.

Research on youth ageing out and transitioning to independent living has been limited. However, both research and anecdotes highlight the unique difficulties that young people who have aged out of foster care and residential settings face (Curry and Abrams, 2014; MassLive.com, 2019). The impact of transitional instability during and after residential life represents a particular challenge for LGBTQIA+ youth when it comes to finding community.

Considering Intersectionality

What does it mean to identify as LGBTQIA+? What does it mean to identify as a person of colour? What is the impact of defining one's gender? How about one's nationality or ethnic group? I could continue with these types of questions. The point is that, as therapists, it is important not to think about these types of questions individually but rather together, like woven pieces, overlapping to form another layer of self-identity, especially in relation to how one may be treated in one's society. In the beginning of my training, I often thought about various identities as separate from each other, not necessarily impacting each other—much more importantly, the broader impact of these intersecting identities on residents' experience of the world around them.

One observation was a difference in how residents formed attachments with peers and staff, especially LGBTQIA+ residents. I noted that some LGBTQIA+ youth remained more detached from their peers and staff, while some formed strong bonds with staff rather than with peers. At first, I attributed that to the lack of certainty of their own length of stay and that of their peers—and that thought is not necessarily incorrect. After all, some youths did not believe they would be in residential care for long and may have decided to keep their distance. Meanwhile, those who had been in residence long term may have preferred to maintain the bonds they had already established with other long-term residents and/or staff. I thought that these attachments and detachments may have contributed to times of perceived group disharmony. I equally noted that residents who identified as belonging to multiple communities (or identities), e.g., being black, transgender, and differently abled, seemed to have the hardest time connecting with peers and, especially, staff (who were predominantly white and female). At that time, I wondered why. What I had not considered was the impact of intersectionality, the interplay of individual biopsychosocial and economic backgrounds in how one experiences and is experienced in the world, on finding a sense of community. This impact may be easily missed if we think of working with youths who identify as LGBTQIA+ as a monolith.

LGBTQIA+ is an umbrella term under which a diverse group of people gather and are gathered. However, being under the same umbrella does not equate with having the same or similar life experiences or even the desire to share space with each other. Research has shown that within the LGBTQIA+ community, various forms of prejudice and discrimination are experienced by those who have intersectional identities (Balsam et al., 2011). Within the LGBTQIA+ youth community, the situation should not be expected to be different. LGBTQIA+ youth should not be expected to have the same life experiences, or to understand each other, or be accepting of each other—it would be ideal if they were, but such a position would not be reflective of U.S. society (Harvard T.H. Chan School of Public Health, Robert Wood Johnson Foundation and National Public Radio, 2018). However, it is important for LGBTQIA+ youth inside and outside of residential settings to find community.

Within the LGBTQIA+ community, there is still a prevalence of creating a family of choice, although there are more members maintaining bonds with their families of origin (Hull and Ortyl, 2019). For those without support from their families of origin, establishing and maintaining a family of choice can be vital to their overall well-being. Jackson Levin et al. (2020) states that LGBTQIA+ individuals with families of choice rely on them to assist with navigating healthcare needs as well as embodying the role of family. For LGBTQIA+ youth in residential settings, especially those who have been there long term, creating bonds in and out of their programmes may be vital to a smoother transition once they leave.

For arts therapies professionals, part of the work that can be done is addressing the theme of finding community, especially within a group therapy context. The focus can be on developing individual and group work that helps LGBTQIA+ youth. For example, tasks that deal with the following topics:

1 Recognise the importance of the space/place they are currently in,
2 Identify the shared interests and values that they have with others within that space,
3 Find ways to create and take action as a community to improve the community,
4 Learn more about each other and form ties, and
5 Confront and resolve biases that may hinder the expression of diversity within the community.

If these topics can be addressed in all forms of therapy, if one is working as part of a treatment team, then much good can be done for clients and the team. Building a team awareness of the intersectionality and addressing intersectionality in both regular talk therapy and in arts therapies are important in improving treatment care for clients.

One of the tasks that I used to address this theme was using materials from popular culture. At that time, that meant using films, documentaries, news and magazine articles, advertisements, etc. I used these materials to appeal to and build on group knowledge, i.e., it was likely that most residents were familiar with these materials. The topics covered varied, from body image to bullying to sexual orientation to misogyny and so on. My choices were informed by the stage of the group development, an understanding of the individual residents, and overall treatment goals.

A Note On Using Literature & Media

In tackling the theme of finding community, I found that films, in particular, fostered self-expression and more open conversations and allowed for residents to take on or try to understand different viewpoints (Dumitrache, 2014; Marsick, 2009). Having residents work together in small groups or pairs on creating collages was also good for improving interpersonal relationships. The collages focused on creating a positive self-image and outlook on the future, a sort of group vision board. In later settings, I used a bibliotherapeutic approach to help residents to build and experience a sense of community. More akin to a book club, residents contributed their suggestions for books that held meaning in their identity development or spoke to their experiences. Unlike the current rapidly growing body of LGBTQIA+ literature and media it was it was far more difficult for LGBTQIA+ youths to find their life stories reflected in literature and the media in the early 2020s, especially positive material.. Back then, residents took joy in imagining a happier future in a family of their own creation, like in the 1989 classic, "Heather Has Two Mommies," by Lesléa Newman.

Given the continuous changes in how we communicate and work as a society, especially amongst young people, it is increasingly important for arts therapies professionals to find ways to utilise new information and communication technology tools, e.g., using social media and networking platforms (Bates et al., 2020; Malchiodi, 2018; Zubala et al., 2021). As we move forward, sharing one's life and doing one's work online will become the norm. As part of the process of change, arts therapies professionals must continue to move forward in improving our knowledge of the spaces in which LGBTQIA+ youths congregate, creating spaces in which they can engage therapeutically, and incorporate digital tools that can facilitate arts therapeutic work.

Addressing the theme of *finding community* can be done using a variety of creative-arts-based approaches, whether working in an individual modality (e.g., art therapy, drama therapy) or in multiple modalities. Ultimately, what is most important is being in tune with the needs of LGBTQIA+ youth, meeting them where they are and helping them to connect with each other and those around them.

Changing Self-identification

Shifting from a question of connecting with others to connecting with one's identity, I found that self-identification changed for some clients. Sometimes change occurred because clients felt more comfortable being themselves because of their new settings and being with other LGBTQIA+ youth. This was especially true for clients who would later identify as being on the trans-spectrum. Conversely, some clients expressed feeling pressured by their peers to maintain an identity that was no longer congruent with their own understanding of themselves.

The American Psychological Association (2021) defined *self-identification* as "the act of construing one's identity in particular terms, usually as a member of a particular group or category ... or as a person with particular traits or attributes." Self-identification is not a static process, but a dynamic experience that changes over the lifespan. Certain associations may remain throughout, but, as one engages the outside world and investigates one's internal world, some aspects of self-identification will likely change (Carter and Marony,

2021; Onorato and Turner, 2004; Oyserman, 2012). In thinking about self-identification as LGBTQIA+, e.g., "I am lesbian," "I am bisexual," I learned that it is important to remember that such identifications may change over time. "I am bisexual" may become "I am lesbian" and vice versa—furthermore, one should not expect that there will always be congruence between identity and behaviour, especially for LGBTQIA+ youth (Rosario et al., 2006).

I found that changes in self-identification could have a profound impact on group therapy in the non-exclusive LGBTQIA+ residential programme. If a group member disclosed a change to their self-identification in or outside of the group, it was usually met with a mix of positive and negative reactions, rarely neutral. For young people who may already find themselves lacking a sense of place and community, the fear of being rejected may be compounded. As a trainee, I focused on empathy-building activities to help groups modulate their responses to disclosure and to create safer space to share disclosures related to gender and sexuality.

Embracing New Modes of Self-expression

Adolescence is a time of exploring the self, as separate from one's family, and beginning the journey towards adulthood. It can be an equally exciting and terrifying time as there is a whirlwind of emotional, mental, and physical changes. Adolescence presents the opportunity for an individual to begin answering the question of identity. Some adolescents' exploration leads them towards identity achievement; for others, the lack of opportunities for exploration, or the process of exploration itself, may prove challenging and lead away from identity achievement (Klym and Cieciuch, 2015). LGBTQIA+ youths are at significant risk of disruptions to their identity development process, if they lack supportive environments in which they can freely express and explore themselves. As noted before, the challenge increases for intersectional LGBTQIA+ youth, who must also tackle the question of their sexual and/or gender identity in relation to their other identities, e.g., race, sex, class, etc. (Leung, 2021). Pelton and Sherry (2008) note that self-expression is important for LGBTQIA+ youth and advocate the use of art therapy in working with them. It is understood that engaging in creative expression can be beneficial to overall wellbeing and Stuckey and Nobel (2010) note that "[t]hrough creativity and imagination, we find our identity and reservoir of healing" (p. 261).

In my experience LGBTQIA+ youth in residential settings were seeking ways to explore the question of who they were and arrive at an answer, while navigating an unfamiliar world. The most prominent emotion displayed by residents I worked with was anger, which was always close to the surface and could erupt at any time in a variety of ways. Helping residents to find more creative ways to channel their emotions, especially anger, was important.

Many of these youths were highly creative, but never had the opportunity to express that creativity. Their voices had often been silenced by those around them. Acting out violently was therefore one way in which some expressed their high levels of distress. Conversely, others would simply withdraw, effectively shutting out the world around them and disconnecting from anything that could cause them additional distress. Meeting and accepting these youths as they presented themselves was important; this involved giving them time and space to find their creative outlet. For some, it was art, others music, crafting, writing, or dance, or a combination of art based practices.. Beyond treatment plans and goals, I saw my primary role as helping them to find their paths towards authentic self-expression.

LGBTQIA+ youth in residential settings will likely need to be introduced to new modes of self-expression. Research indicates that LGBTQIA+ youth are more likely to have come from environments in which they were subjected to abuse (emotionally, physically, and/or sexually) and are more likely to have turned to maladaptive behaviours as coping tools, such as engaging in substance abuse (Choi et al., 2015). Speaking about their feelings and thoughts may be difficult for them. As such, the use of creative arts therapies in their treatment can be vital in helping them learn how to safely express and manage their feelings and thoughts (Huerta, 2018; Riley, 2001).

Bridging the Multicultural Gap

"I thought you were a snob," said one group member, while others nodded in agreement. I smiled when I heard these words. In truth, I was quite shocked that I had been perceived like that by the group when we first met. "Yeah, I mean, you look like us, but you sure don't sound like us," another group member said. With those words, I began to understand a very important lesson: I must always take into consideration the multicultural gap. I realised that I had fallen into the space between myself and my clients, thinking that they would find it easy to relate to me because we were of similar background (being of African descent). And based upon the very frank and unprompted conversation they continued to have with me, they let me know that they, too, had been excited to have someone who looked like me as one of their group therapists—until I spoke. My manner of speaking placed me outside of their world, as someone who could not understand their experiences. With time, their perceptions of me changed. However, the lesson that they taught me on that day remained: as a therapist, it is my job to bridge the gap between myself and my clients.

Every June, for Pride Month, the American Art Therapy Association publishes an article that highlights an aspect of the LGBTQIA+ community in relation to art therapy. In 2018, art therapist Daniel Blausey wrote an article titled "June is Pride Month. Here's what art therapists need to know." In this article, Blausey (2018) highlighted the importance of learning more about the LGBTQIA+ community, especially the terminology used, and to "bring awareness to any conscious or unconscious bias of the art therapist and address the potential impact our attitudes, beliefs, and values have when working with clients" (p. 1).

One of the concerns that LGBTQIA+ youth have when working with therapists is that that person will not understand their concerns or be adequately able to meet their therapeutic needs (Choi et al., 2015; Green et al., 2020). Research has shown that there are benefits to LGBTQIA+ youth when they are in programmes that include staff who are adequately trained in LGBTQIA+ issues (Burwick et al., 2014; Choi et al., 2015; Green et al., 2020; Poirier et al., 2008). As arts therapies professionals we must also take care to broaden our multicultural competency scope in how we approach our work with all groups of people. LGBTQIA+ youth, especially intersectional LGBTQIA+ youth, whether in a residential setting or not, can and will benefit from the tools that arts therapies professionals can provide.

Summary

More recently, the creative arts therapies community has begun addressing the need for information about working with the LGBTQIA+ community (MacWilliam et al., 2019; Whitman and Boyd, 2021). This is a step in a positive direction and indicates a growing awareness. I am hopeful that that awareness will quickly extend to include works focused on LGBTQIA+ youth, especially those who are living in residential settings.

I began this chapter by indicating five themes that emerged while working with LGBTQIA+ youth in residential settings as a graduate student trainee in expressive therapy: social displacement, challenges to finding community, changing self-identification, embracing new modes of self-expression, and bridging the multicultural gap. I have attempted to illustrate how these themes emerged and why they are important to address when working with this population. LGBTQIA+ youth in residential settings stand at a crossroads, trying to make sense of both an old and new reality. They are attempting to find their place in the world while trying to know who they are in relation to others, and seeking ways to safely express themselves because they want to be heard. Arts therapies professionals can make a valuable contribution to processes conducive to empowerment in these young people and contribute to their finding their voice and their path.

References

Addison, D. (1996). Message of Acceptance: "Gay-Friendly" Art Therapy for Homosexual Clients. *Art Therapy: Journal of the American Art Therapy Association*, 13(1), pp. 54–56, DOI: 10.1080/07421656.1996.10759193.

American Psychological Association. (n.d.). Self-identification. In *Dictionary.APA.org*. Retrieved August 7, 2021, from https://dictionary.apa.org/self-identification.

Balsam, K. F., Molina, Y., Beadnell, B., Simoni, J., and Walters, K. (2011). Measuring multiple minority stress: the LGBT People of Color Microaggressions Scale. *Cultural diversity & ethnic minority psychology*, 17(2), pp. 163–174. 10.1037/a0023244

Barbot, B. (2018). Creativity and Self-esteem in Adolescence: A Study of Their Domain-Specific, Multivariate Relationships. *The Journal of Creative Behavior*, 54. 10.1002/jocb.365.

Bates, A., Hobman, T., and Bell, B. T. (2020). "Let Me Do What I Please With It ... Don't Decide My Identity For Me": LGBTQ+ Youth Experiences of Social Media in Narrative Identity Development. *Journal of Adolescent Research*, 35(1), pp. 51–83.

Blausey, D. (2018). June is Pride Month. Here's what art therapists need to know. *American Art Therapy Association*. Retrieved August 17, 2021, https://arttherapy.org/blog-pride-month-what-art-therapists-should-know/

Brody, R. (2013). Becoming Visible: An Art Therapy Support Group for Isolated Low-Income Lesbians. *Art Therapy: Journal of the American Art Therapy Association*, 13, pp. 20–30. 10.1080/07421656.1996.10759189.

Burwick, A., Oddo, V., Durso, L., Friend, D., and Gates, G. (2014). Identifying and Serving LGBTQ Youth: Case Studies of Runaway and Homeless Youth Program Grantees. *Mathematica Policy Research*. Retrieved June 2, 2021, https://aspe.hhs.gov/reports/identifying-serving-lgbtq-youth-case-studies-runaway-homeless-youth-programme-grantees-0.

Cambridge Dictionary. (n.d.). Displacement. In *Dictionary.Cambridge.org* dictionary. Retrieved August 10, 2021, from https://dictionary.cambridge.org/dictionary/english/displacement.

Carter, M. and Marony, J. (2021). Examining Self-Perceptions of Identity Change in Person, Role, and Social Identities. *Current Psychology*, 40. 10.1007/s12144-018-9924-5.

Choi, S. K., Wilson, B. D. M., Shelton, J., and Gates, G. (2015). *Serving Our Youth 2015: The Needs and Experiences of Lesbian, Gay, Bisexual, Transgender, and Questioning Youth Experiencing Homelessness*. Los Angeles: The Williams Institute with True Colors Fund.

Commonwealth of Massachusetts. (2018, September 1). *Youth in State Care*. https://www.mass.gov/handbook/youth-in-state-care

Curry, S. and Abrams, L. (2014). Housing and Social Support for Youth Aging Out of Foster Care: State of the Research Literature and Directions for Future Inquiry. *Child and Adolescent Social Work Journal*, 32. 10.1007/s10560-014-0346-4.

Dumitrache, S. (2014). The Effects of a Cinema-therapy Group on Diminishing Anxiety in Young People. *Procedia - Social and Behavioral Sciences*, 127, pp. 717–721. 10.1016/j.sbspro.2014.03.342.

Gilroy, A. (2006). *Art Therapy, Research and Evidence-Based Practice*. London: SAGE Publications.

Green, A. E., Price-Feeney, M., and Dorison, S. (2020). *Breaking Barriers to Quality Mental Health Care for LGBTQ Youth*. New York, New York: The Trevor Project.

Harvard T.H. Chan School of Public Health, Robert Wood Johnson Foundation and National Public Radio. (2018). Discrimination in America: Final Report. *Harvard.edu*. Retrieved August 7, 2021, from https://cdn1.sph.harvard.edu/wp-content/uploads/sites/94/2018/01/NPR-RWJF-HSPH-Discrimination-Final-Summary.pdf

Hall, J. A., Kearney, M. W., and Xing, C. (2019). Two tests of social displacement through social media use. *Information, Communication & Society*, 22(10), pp. 1396–1413, DOI: 10.1080/1369118X.2018.1430162.

Huerta, T. (2018). *Use of the Creative Arts Therapies and Creative Interventions with LGBTQ Individuals: Speaking out from Silence a Literature Review*. [Unpublished doctoral dissertation]. Lesley University.

Hull, K. E. and Ortyl, T. A. (2019). Conventional and Cutting-Edge: Definitions of Family in LGBT Communities. *Sexuality Research and Social Policy*, 16(1), pp. 31–43. 10.1007/s13178-018-0324-2.

Jackson Levin, N., Kattari, S. K., Piellusch, E. K., and Watson, E. (2020). "We Just Take Care of Each Other": Navigating 'Chosen Family' in the Context of Health, Illness, and the Mutual Provision of Care amongst Queer and Transgender Young Adults. *International Journal of environmental research and public health*, 17(19), p. 7346. 10.3390/ijerph17197346

Katz-Wise, S. L., Rosario, M., and Tsappis, M. (2016). Lesbian, Gay, Bisexual, and Transgender Youth and Family Acceptance. *Pediatric clinics of North America*, 63(6), pp. 1011–1025. 10.1016/j.pcl.2016.07.005.

Klym, M. and Cieciuch, J. (2015). The Early Identity Exploration Scale measures initial exploration in breadth during early adolescence. *Frontiers in Psychology*. 10.3389/fpsyg.2015.00533.

Leung, E. (2021). Thematic Analysis of My "Coming Out" Experiences Through an Intersectional Lens: An Autoethnographic Study. *Frontiers in Psychology*. 10.3389/fpsyg.2021.654946

MacQueen, K., McLellan-Lemal, E., Metzger, D., Kegeles, S., Strauss, R., Scotti, R., Blanchard, L., and Trotter II, R. (2001). What Is Community? An Evidence-Based Definition for Participatory Public Health. *American Journal of Public Health*, 91. pp. 1929–1938. 10.2105/AJPH.91.12.1929.

MacWilliam, B., Harris, B. T., Trottier D. G., and Long, K. (Eds.) (2019). *Creative Arts Therapies and the LGBTQ Community*. London & Philadelphia: Jessica Kingsley Publishers.

Malchiodi, C. A. (2018, February 18). Art Therapy and Social Media. *PsychologyToday.com*. Retrieved August 7, 2021, https://www.psychologytoday.com/intl/blog/arts-and-health/201802/art-therapy-and-social-media

Marsick, E. (2009). *Cinematherapy with Preadolescents Experiencing Parental Divorce: A Collective Case Study*. [Unpublished doctoral dissertation]. Cambridge, Massachusetts: Lesley University.

Massachusetts Society for the Prevention of Cruelty to Children. (2005). 18 and Out: Life After Foster Care in Massachusetts. Retrieved August 7, 2021, https://www.chapa.org/sites/default/files/qwert_16.pdf

https://www.masslive.com/news/2019/04/theres-no-way-for-us-to-learn-how-to-live-foster-children-who-age-out-of-care-suffer-later-in-life.html

Merriam-Webster. (n.d.). Social. In the *Merriam-Webster.com* dictionary. Retrieved August 10, 2021, from https://www.merriam-webster.com/dictionary/social.

Morton, M. H., Dworsky, A., and Samuels, G. M. (2017). *Missed opportunities: Youth homelessness in America. National estimates*. Chicago, IL: Chapin Hall at the University of Chicago.

Onorato, R. and Turner, J. (2004). Fluidity in the Self-Concept: The Shift from Personal to Social Identity. *European Journal of Social Psychology*, 34, pp. 257–278. 10.1002/ejsp.195.

Oyserman, D. (2012). Self-Concept and Identity. *ResearchGate.com*. Retrieved August 10, 2021, https://www.researchgate.net/publication/280230936_Self-Concept_and_Identity.

Pelton-Sweet, L. and Sherry, A. (2008). Coming out through art: A review of art therapy with LGBT clients. *Art Therapy: Journal of the American Art Therapy Association*, 25. 10.1080/07421656.2008.10129546.

Poirier, J. M., Francis, K. B., Fisher, S. K., Williams- Washington, K., Goode, T. D., and Jackson, V. H. (2008). *Practice Brief 1: Providing Services and Supports for Youth Who Are Lesbian, Gay, Bisexual, Transgender, Questioning, Intersex, or Two-Spirit*. Washington, DC: National Center for Cultural Competence, Georgetown University Center for Child and Human Development.

Riley, S. (2001). Art therapy with adolescents. *The Western Journal of Medicine*, 175(1), pp. 54–57. 10.1136/ewjm.175.1.54.

Rosario, M., Schrimshaw, E. W., Hunter, J., and Braun, L. (2006). Sexual identity development among gay, lesbian, and bisexual youths: consistency and change over time. *Journal of Sex Research*, 43(1), pp. 46–58. 10.1080/00224490609552298

Smith, D. (2010). Social Fluidity and Social Displacement. *The Sociological Review*, 58(4), pp. 680–698.

Stuckey, H. L. and Nobel, J. (2010). The connection between art, healing, and public health: a review of current literature. *American Journal of Public Health*, 100(2), pp. 254–263. 10.2105/AJPH.2008.156497.

Whitman, J. S. and Boyd, C. J. (Eds.). (2021). *Homework Assignments and Handouts for LGBTQ+ Clients: A mental health and counseling handbook*. New York and London: Routledge.

Wing Sue, D. and Sue, D. (2008). *Counseling the culturally diverse: Theory and practice* (5th ed.). Hoboken, New Jersey: John Wiley & Sons, Inc.

Yarhouse, M., Sides, J., and Page, C. (2018). The Complexities of Multicultural Competence with LGBT+ Populations: An Evaluation of Current Status and Future Directions. 10.1007/978-3-319-78997-2_23.

Youth.gov (n.d.). *Homelessness and Housing*, https://youth.gov/youth-topics/lgbtq-youth/homelessness.

Zubala, A., Kennell, N., and Hackett, S. (2021). Art Therapy in the Digital World: An Integrative Review of Current Practice and Future Directions. *Frontiers in Psychology*, 12, p. 595536. 10.3389/fpsyg.2021.600070.

Chapter 11

The Leelah Play

Dov Blum-Yazdi

Introduction

Leelah is a Sanskrit word that describes world creation as a rhythmic play in which the Gods engage in endless cycles. I called Leelah Play (Blum-Yazdi, 2019) a dramatic/dramaturgic therapeutic method that uses play for therapy, combining theories of drama with classical psychoanalytic concepts. The Leelah Play consists of two parts. The Leelah Play Paradigm is a theory that redefines terms such as power relationship, freedom, and identity of the playing person in therapy. The Leelah—Play for Itself is an application of the Leelah Play Paradigm, just one of many possible ways for applying it. The Leelah—Play for Itself is based on undirected role-play within the frame of a long-term narrative. This model suggests a therapeutic process of non-intervention, an autonomous and self-healing work led by the players themselves, where the play stands for itself.

In this chapter, firstly, I will describe the different levels of intervention; subsequently, I will present the Leelah model as a non-intervention role-play therapy; finally, I will show some vignettes of an application of the model with a group of young people. I consider spontaneous, natural child play the most important form of play; thus, my work with young people and adults leads there as Nietzsche (2001) declared: 'The maturity of man, that means, to have reacquired the seriousness that one had as a child at play.' (ibid, p. 101).

Pendzik (2006) claims that drama therapy invariably occurs inside a Dramatic Reality, which can be considered a major therapeutic intervention: 'teaching someone how to create a dramatic reality constitutes in itself an intervention' (ibid, p. 278). Johnson (1992) describes various degrees of involvement of the drama therapists within the dramatic reality, ranging from being a witness, director, side-coach, leader, or guide to a shaman.

Pitruzzella (2004) explains that the person in drama therapy must be aware of her engagement and disengagement and find her Aesthetic Distance from the drama (ibid, pp. 99–100). Following this, Aesthetic Distance in Leelah means that the therapist should avoid unnecessary interventions; because therapeutic interventions might serve normalisation rather than people's needs.

DOI: 10.4324/9781003265610-12

The Leelah approach distinguishes between Naive[1] Intervention and Clinical Intervention; the former is related to the presence and existence of the therapist in the here and now, and the latter concerns the actions made by the therapist in order to bypass or break the player's defences or transfer information about the player that the therapist apparently knows better than the player itself. I will discuss the Clinical Intervention by drawing a spectrum of intervention levels and locate Leelah among other models that use play in therapy.

At one pole of the spectrum, we can put theories and models in which the therapist holds a dominant place, where intervention and interpretation are prominent, and where play serves as a tool for purposes not inherent to the play itself. In the middle, we have theories and models in which the therapist is located in the background. His intervention accompanies the player, offers different interpretations, and uses only necessary intervention.

Finally, at the other pole, we find models where the therapist allows natural processes of self-healing; play occurs spontaneously and for its own sake. Thus, the therapist has various levels of intervention at his disposal, including non-interventional therapeutic action (Figure 11.1).

Leelah defines as **Biased-Intervention** a prominent action performed by a 'clever' therapist, which affects the player directly or indirectly to lead to structural and perceptual changes in his worldview or personality. This action bypasses Defence Mechanism; it is done either openly or discreetly and can be done verbally or through play. 'The significant moment is that at which the child surprises himself ... not the moment of my clever interpretation ...' notes Winnicott (1975, p. 51). In Biased-Interventions, the intervention level is high, and the Aesthetic Distance level is low.

Leelah defines phenomenological action as any non-intrusive act that allows the player to develop the play in his own unique way, based on the acceptance at face value of his worldview and personality structure. Therefore, this action will not be concrete and focused but rather broad and dynamic, respecting Defence Mechanism. 'Psychotherapy of a deep-going kind may be done without interpretative work' emphasises Winnicott (1975, p.50). In phenomenological action, the intervention level is low, and the Aesthetic Distance level is high (Figure 11.2).

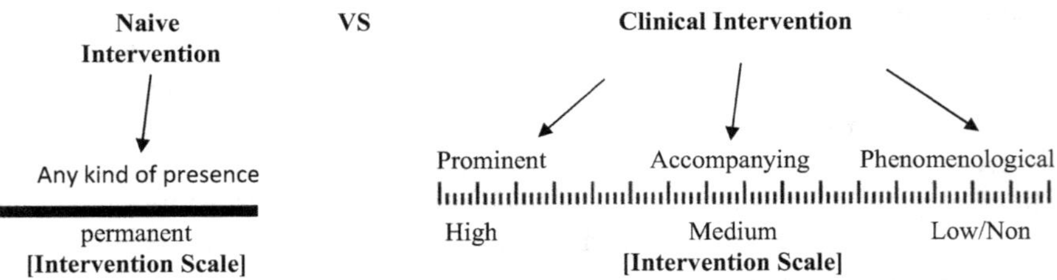

Figure 11.1 Naive intervention vs clinical intervention.

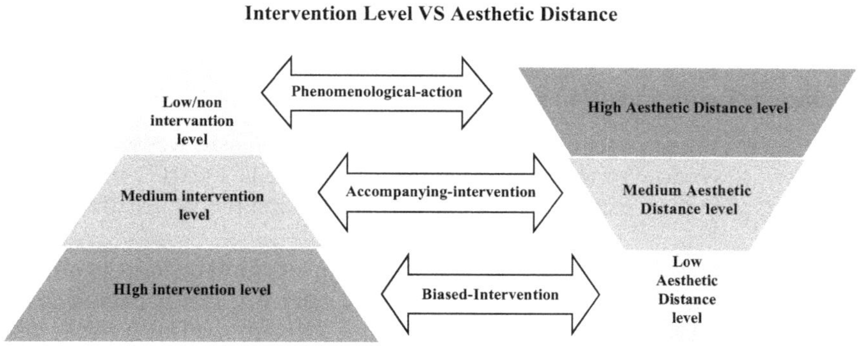

Figure 11.2 Intervention level vs aesthetic distance.

Prominent intervention models

The classic Kleinian theory is an example of a play model and theory where the therapist is very dominant, intervening and interpreting tendentiously. Klein (1959) claimed that the status of play is equivalent to that of free associations that represent the subconscious; therefore, she used to interpret children's playful activities: 'the elements of children's play, which correspond to those associations, afford a view of its latent meaning.' (ibid, p. 43).

Similarly, Johnson (1992) describes the Developmental Transformations method as improvising continuous transformation of embodied encounters in a Playspace.

According to Gideon Zehavi (personal communication, 2022), 'the therapist takes on the role of "play object" and actively interacts with the client drawing upon numerous dramatic intervention techniques'. As mentioned earlier, the therapist's position can range from being a witness, director, side coach, shaman, and leader. The therapist 'can also act as a knowledgeable guide ... While similar in function to the leader position, the therapist as a guide is allowed a greater degree of centrality ... "Therapist as subject" ... actually becomes the major focus of the drama' (Johnson, 1992, p. 115).

Classical psychodrama is also characterised by the prominent presence and intervention of the psychodramatist. In this technique, spontaneous play can occur only after the therapist bypasses the patient's Defence Mechanisms. The psychodramatist acts as a theatre director: after he chooses the protagonist, he is in charge of navigating the psychodrama, encourages the patient to expose himself, and overcomes his resistance. In Mary's study case, Moreno (1944) lists an 'Index of techniques' (Ibid, p. 324). The eighth is Hypno-drama: 'Mary resists acting with William as the John-substitute ... The director, assuming a technique of heightened authority and aggression towards the subject, orders Mary step by step what to do. Mary follows directions as if under the influence of hypnotic suggest' (Ibid, p. 325).

Accompanying intervention models

While, according to psychoanalytic theory, play is similar to free associations and opens a window to the subconscious, in Pitruzzella's (2017) humanistic approach, play is an expression of the authentic potential of creativity:

> At the core of dramatherapy, there is a form of humanism, a profound respect for the other, whom we always consider not just a person to be helped, but a herald of potential creativity. This humanism informs our approach, as well as the values that underlie it (ibid, p. 136).

Here are some examples of models wherein the therapist is perceived as allowing, intervenes carefully, and uses accompanying intervention.

One of the main aims of Landy's (1996) Role Method is to foster people's ability to expand their role repertoire by experimenting with a large spectrum of roles. Landy's model poses that no role exists in isolation from the others, and each role has complementary, contrasting, expanding, or diminishing aspects. Building each Role, a Counter-Role is implicit, and a Guide can emerge as a mediator between the two: 'The role method in drama in drama therapy ... attempts to further systematise what is views as the primary component of healing ...' (ibid. p. 45–46).

Dramatic Resonances (Pendzik, 2008) and psychotherapeutic playback theatre (Kowalsky et al., 2019) are techniques that can be applied as an accompanying intervention used in group settings. These methods are based on participants' creative responses within dramatic reality to an input posed from outside dramatic reality. The information may be a member's personal experience (memory, dream, etc.) or a non-personal narrative (tale, text, etc.). These approaches have a robust ritualistic style and integrate elements from various sources.

Phenomenological/non-intervention models

The phenomenological approach (Husserl, 2012) argues that to 'see' we must pause our knowledge of things from the past (Phenomenological Reduction). Phenomenology, literally the science of appearances, is a systematic description of conscious awareness, which results in grasping the essence of phenomena. Moreover, it helps us in setting aside our usual assumptions and biases. This approach avoids prescription, interpretation, and intervention.

Mook (2003) explains that sand-play therapy through a phenomenological approach helps our brain collect details and not decipher them. The patient is invited to give an opinion on various qualities on stage, such as perspective and choice of details about the characters. The play is free of judgement. This approach is not interpretative and strives to describe the phenomenon from its own qualities rather than from previous frames of interpretation. In other words, 'The less the therapist knows, the more the patient will know' (Heller, personal communication, 2022).

Jennings (1995) claims that we should be loyal to the metaphorical expressions made by the patient and not force control by interpreting them. 'Our need to explain and interpret is more about our own feelings of anxiety than our client's' (ibid, p. 37).

We should stay with not knowing and allow meaning to be discovered with time. Analysing the story and interpreting the inner, symbolic material of the patient is not part of the role of the drama therapist; this is a claim made by the Sesame method, a British approach to therapy through drama and movement (Hougham, 2006). Like Jennings, this method is metaphorical work. It does not intervene and is based on the assumption that difficulties are indirectly resolved through distancing. The integration process and healing occur over time by themselves.

The therapeutic approach of Carl Rogers (2007) assumes that the client is the expert in himself and can find solutions to his problems. The therapist's role is to allow the natural expression of the client, and the only intervention is repeating his words. According to Rogers, one of the superior qualities of the therapist is complete acceptance of the client as they are and the ability of the therapist to be unmasked. According to the humanistic approach of Axline (1964) to play therapy, based on Rogers, the therapist does not interpret but allows space and mirrors the child's behaviour. Some of the basic principles are accepting of the child for who he is, not directing the behaviour of the child; the therapist does not attempt to advance therapy; the therapist determines only the necessary boundaries for anchoring the therapy in reality and passing the responsibility on the relationship to the child.

Similar to Axline, Erikson (1993) insists on un-intervention in the child's play: 'The most obvious condition is that ... any kind of sudden interruption does not disturb the unfolding of his play intentions, wherever they may be' (ibid, p. 222).

Considering these ideas, Leelah Play is placed at the edge of the spectrum where the therapist avoids interventions, and play is not used as a tool to bypass Defence Mechanism. Instead, the goal of therapy is to create a playful space that is healing in itself, with a noticeable Aesthetic Distance. In Leelah, play can occur only when it has no purpose outside of itself.

Presenting 'Leelah – Play for Itself'

The model, 'Leelah – Play for Itself,' (Blum-Yazdi, 2014), relies on a storyline where the players portray set characters. The therapist suggests a narrative background and provides general rules. The rest of the plot is devised interactively by the characters that develop during the play. Few scenes are happening simultaneously, creating a playful space. This space is open and unpredictable since each character's actions depend on the autonomous decisions of the player and on the developing relationships among characters. The model has two major sources of inspiration: the way of working through the autonomous group process was inspired by the Greek *Polis,* while the way of working through roles and storylines by the game Dungeons & Dragons (D&D).

The play concepts

In his book, Homo Ludens, Huizinga (2014) claims that play is a free activity that serves no purpose, neither by nature nor by society. Defining the play Winnicott (1975) emphasises the state of deep concentration: 'the content does not matter. What matters is the near-withdrawal state ... the concentration ... The playing child inhabits an area that cannot be easily left, nor can it easily admit intrusions' (ibid, p. 51). Next to Winnicott, Erikson underscores the lightness of play:

> When a man plays, he must intermingle with things and people in a similarly uninvolved and light fashion. He must do something he has chosen without being compelled by urgent interests or impelled by strong passion; he must feel entertained and free of any fear or hope of serious consequences (Erikson 1993, p. 212).

Therefore, here are some of the basic concepts I have established.

Basic assumptions

Suchness play

Play in its ultimate state of healing, in its simplicity, play in itself. The essence or nature of playing before ideas or words. A creative activity, free of external demands and unrelated to reward, winning, or achievements. It is not an object of projective material of the unconscious: suchness play is the substance itself.

Play collapse situations

An entirely therapeutic play situation occurs when there are no: 1. Goals outside of play; 2. Audience watching the play; 3. Interpretation and/or an aware connection to life. If one or more of these three features happens, the play is 'abused' for the sake of other things and can no longer be considered a play.

Self-healing

It happens within Suchness Play when the play is spontaneous, when the player is offered safe and appropriate conditions, without competition or blame, no matter his intentions, and when play occurs autonomously.

Play frame

The therapeutic work is done through the storyline and character portrayal—the model is compatible with the notion Jennings (1999) has of the balance required in therapeutic work through drama between the element of 'ritual' and the element of 'risk'; the frame and the ritual create security, predictability, and knowability. They act as a container for development, journey, and adventure. The risk means going on an adventure where everything can be new and different, being open to a different outlook beyond the known and familiar. In the play, everyone portrays roles, including the therapist, so there are no witnesses or audience.

Aletheaic play space (APS)

Describing the absorption quality of play, Gersie (1987) claims: 'Interruption are experienced as an intense violation of privacy for they disturb the pattern of inner activity ...' (Ibid, p. 52). In order to play with devotion, we need to feel both safe and safeguarded against unwanted intrusion ...' (p. 46). Leelah defines the dramatic reality as Aletheaic Play Space (APS) to protect the player's play.

APS is a vast dramatic space that contains:

Organic Play Space (OPS), which is meant for the player alone, allowing a withdrawal state of deep concentration, free from any interventions.

Transitional Play Space (TPS), similar to the Winnicottian transitional space, is meant for the therapist alone, from which one can reach insights and an outer observation of the play. The therapist's external reflection occurs only after the play and never during it. The space between parent and baby illustrates APS. For the baby, it is an actual space in itself (OPS), while for the parent, it is also a space for experiencing and outer observation (TPS). (Figure 11.3)

The play course[2]

The Avatar

Leelah uses the term Avatar to describe the player's role. The Leelah therapy is directed to the Avatar, not to the player, meaning the Avatar is the one who gets the therapy. Leelah claims that the Avatar affects the player

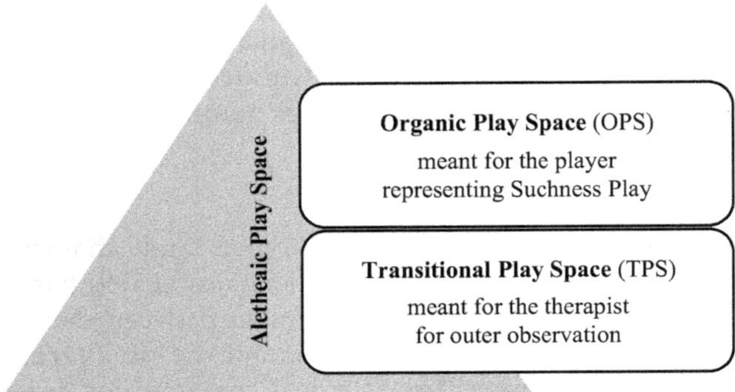

Figure 11.3 Aletheaic play space (APS).

because the player and his Avatar have a mutual relationship. Thus, eventually, the therapy involves the player indirectly. The Leelah core clinical aspect is working with the Developmental Sequences of the Avatar (see Illustration section).

In order to work indirectly with healing metaphors, the player must avoid blurring the mental line between him and his Avatar. The Avatar must be distinguished from the player. It should have a different personality, name, and acquaintances, and a distinctive appearance, profession, and biography. The player should keep a mental distance from his Avatar and not identify with it. Making direct connections or interpretations between those two kills the healing metaphor.

Creating the Avatar is happening one time at the beginning of the first session. It occurs shortly, spontaneously, randomly, without thinking, using standard dramatherapy tools. Leelah's goal is to experience a whole and deep process of therapeutic play. Therefore, all participants make a commitment to stick to their Avatar. Since it is a long-term therapy, we stay with the same Avatar for a few months. It doesn't matter how many transformations the Avatar goes through a narrative and a storyline is developing anyway amongst the changes. During the sessions, people keep playing the Avatar from the beginning to the end. There are two ways to get out of the Avatar during the session: A short Exit and a Long Exit to an introspective space.

Participating in the play doesn't require acting skills. Leelah suits those who are afraid of role-playing games. It allows gentle, quiet, calm, and pleasant role play. There is no need to be a funny, successful, or talented player. There's no such thing as a player that acts up or fails to function correctly. The only request is to be attentive and loyal to your feelings and play with them. During the sessions, we keep the MBP (Mind, Body, Possessions) rules; players act respectfully towards one another, keeping each other's privacy, physical boundaries, and possessions intact.

Self-organisation and feedback

Since all the various characters exist in the same world, Leelah creates a complex system where each character's decisions affect the others. Thus, the Leelah plot of the game is a complex system and a collective, non-linear creation of the player, which surprises even the maker of the game himself.

Lahad (2000) explains that sometimes he invites his supervisees to think of the group as a system or as an organisation, such as a factory or a circus or a place such as a central station or an airport. Self-organisation is a quality of the systems identified by the new sciences of complexity (Capra, 2013). Applied to the group process, it implies a natural, independent healing capability of the group.

Its basic assumption is that small changes in the primary connections between group members may lead to broader changes in the group as a whole. Accordingly, one of the ground rules of the model is the principle of feedback. Feedback in Leelah is a process in which information regarding the outcome of an event of the play affects the development or the interruption of the event itself or of another event. Through continuous reciprocal feedback, the group receives information from its own activity, which allows them to correct and rebalance the system. The system's self-rebalancing occurs naturally when the group has a stable and safe APS. Any intervention of the therapist is unnecessary. Feedback at the player level is the measure by which the player learns about the play from the play itself, not needing any form of interpretation.

Play beats

The play begins in an imaginary town and has three repetitive beats; it starts individually and gets wider gradually and circular/spirally. The therapist is in charge of the play frame and repeatedly takes the townspeople through the beats while the townspeople control the plot and the content. The first beat is **'Personal Stage,'** and it is Pre/Pro-Interaction. The beat goals are to create a safe personal place and a self-reflection area for the persona. The play starts and ends there, privately. The second beat is **'Social Stage,'** the beat goals are to create different social circles: guild circle, neighbourhood circle, et cetera, and practising the persona skills. The town people are invited to guild meetings and to wander in the town alleys. The third beat is the **'Worldwide Context Stage,'** the beat goal is to enable a spacious awareness which happens during the town guild assembly. Those three beats help Avatars to go through developmental psychological stages (Figure 11.4).

Like the players, the therapist sticks to his Avatar and acts through it during the play, so there is no external eye watching it and no audience. After the cool-down, the group sits in a circle to process and close the play. The players speak about their Avatars in the third person, avoiding making any

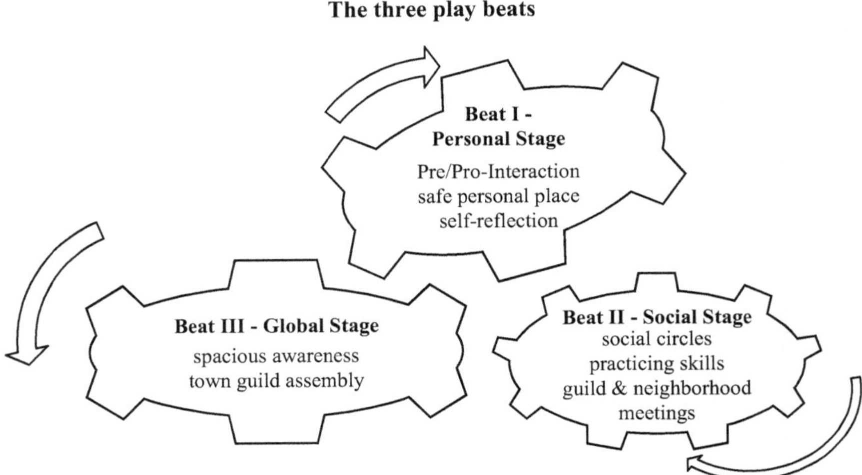

Figure 11.4 The three beats.

connections or interpretations to themselves. The therapeutic process echoes in the players' lives independently and naturally, without analysis or biased interpretation of the story and the role. One of Leelah's clinical cores is working with Developmental Sequences. In the next section, I will explain how it works.

Developmental sequences

Meet Ferro and Portofino town

Ferro is an Italian man in his early 30s, a member of the Strozzi dynasty. He was once part of the European aristocracy. He was born in Florence to a Christian mother and a Jewish father and played a key role in cultivating the 'new music' of his city. He was a member of Count Giovanni de Bardi's Florentine Camerata. As an aristocrat, Ferro led a happy and vital life and was as free as a bird: he never cared much about finding a spouse or building a family. But Ferro's luck ran out. Being a reckless young musician, he lost all his money and, as a result, forfeited his noble title.

Penniless and broken-hearted, Ferro set out wandering and ended up living in a humble little neighbourhood of a small town called Portofino, next to six other neighbours: *the town elder*—a nameless old man of questionable sanity; *Mr Jacob*—a skilled and sentimental construction worker; *Rory*—a hard-working and optimistic sheriff who is exasperated by his townsfolk; *Julietta*—an elitist and alienated artist who longs for companionship; *David*—a dark attorney who is looking for the light; *Sansey*—a graceful and light-hearted stylist who gets on everybody's nerves. In this town, Ferro works as the king's messenger and earns his living with menial tasks such as lighting the streetlamps or handing out tea; he is even known to beg.

All these Avatars are at the starting point of the fascinating journey of a drama therapy group, which lasted four months. It was a group of young people, mainly in their early 20s, and counted seven members, including me as a therapist, while Ferro was my Avatar. It was a heterogeneous group; there were secular Jews, religious Jews, Druze Arabs, and new Christian immigrants who converted to Judaism; the proportion of men to women was almost equal, and some members played a character of the opposite gender.

Meet the town elder and Mr Jacob

After our visit to the town is over, and we leave our Avatars behind, we engage in sharing. Sharing can be performed through speech or writing, with each player discussing their Avatar in the third person in order to distinguish themselves from the character they portrayed fully. Notice the richness and depth with which one of the players describes her Avatar, the town elder:

> The town elder is over 100 years old. He is twice widowed and has no contact with his children. He doesn't remember either his name or his past. He is always surrounded by birds, which he generously feeds with the best millet. His shack is located by the river and is covered with branches and leaves. Physically, he is weak, hard of hearing, and low functioning. He loves when people come and visit him and listen to the fairy tales he tells. He ekes out a living by running an old antique shop. Fortunately for him, almost no one ever buys anything because the objects he sells are like his family. Each tool has its own story, soul and secret. He talks to them and keeps them safe as if they were babies. The townspeople respect him but also make fun of him—they cannot live with him and cannot live without him.
>
> On the one hand, he is a symbol of the town's past; just like a monument, the history of the place is literally engraved in him. On the other hand, he refuses to fit in and keeps disrupting the order. Let us now meet Mr Jacob and consider his interaction with the town elder.
>
> This is how the player depicted Mr Jacob:
>
> *Mr Jacob is the town's older resident; he is over 60 years old and a healthy man. He has been married for many years and, much like his relationship with the other townspeople, he maintains a respectful, although not intimate, relationship with his wife. He has two grown-up daughters who have moved out; one is married. He spends most of his time working in*

construction and has no hobbies. He leads a simple and modest life, likes to look at the town's buildings, chats with his neighbours, visits his good old friend, the town elder, reads a newspaper and smokes his pipe. After a long day spent around the town, he prefers to stay home and have a good bowl of soup alone. He is a very practical and pragmatic person. His notion is that 'it's 'fine,' that everyone is okay, and he does not dig any deeper than that. Even though he is a rather typical example of masculine indifference, he has some emotional qualities as a sentimental type.

This is what the player said about Mr Jacob's exploits during the sharing. Note how absorbed and devoted the players are to their Avatar:

One morning, Mr Jacob went out to meet some of his neighbours. He was cool and distant, as usual. He met an old friend with whom he had spent part of his childhood—the nameless elder. Jacob is supportive and sympathetic towards the elder out of respect for his senility. Mr Jacob exchanged a few words with Sansey, the stylist and Sheriff Rory and tried to figure out Julietta, the artist's true nature. His old friend sold him a bowl of soup and, in exchange, asked for his hat. On his part, Mr Jacob did not intend to give up his precious hat and therefore offered his friend a new one he would make for next week. Julietta, who was present when the deal was made, tried to cause a fight between the two by claiming that Mr Jacob was taking advantage of the elder's senility and did not intend to deliver the promised hat. Because Mr Jacob did have the elder's best interests at heart, this confused and hurt him, and he could not understand why he is being accused.

At this point, the player reported the collapse of her Avatar:

I felt hurt, wronged, misunderstood and that I wasn't Mr Jacob anymore but myself. I felt a need to turn to the person who played Julietta, share my feelings with him and ask him why he accused me.

This is a moment in which the Avatar, Mr Jacob, broke down because he merged with the player, who adhered to the values that guided her real-life conduct. In *Leelah*, players are free to play with, explore, and revisit their sets of values. The player's need to adhere to values such as 'keeping the peace' or 'decency' is part of her everyday conduct and, as such, is unrelated to the roleplay. It, therefore, represents a process of self-disciplining on her part. Bringing this value to bear on the Avatar constitutes the kind of social regulation that we seek to avoid. The *Leelah* model creates a playful space that invites us to be free and act in ways that are not necessarily considered ethical.

Through Ferro, the therapist, I invite Mr Jacob to conduct his inquiry in-play. Off-play, I invite the player to resist identifying herself with her Avatar and to allow herself to feel hurt, offended, and confused, as well as to express these feelings within the town setting. Avatars are allowed to feel hurt, angry or betrayed. All emotions are welcome, and there is no desire to keep to positive emotions, as dictated by society. Healing may occur precisely through the encounter with diverse emotions and by working these through by means of the Avatar—and not by avoiding them and defining them as irrelevant to our development.

Developmental sequences—core clinical aspect

Let us go back to the theoretical aspects. The way in which Avatars are accompanied in Leelah's play is informed by an awareness of the power relations between therapist and patient and derived from the paradigm's definition of the identity of the playing subject in therapy.

The Leelah paradigm draws on the triple spiral (Triskelion, an ancient Celtic symbol) as a form of the psyche of the Avatar. Each of these three spirals is a staircase spiral (Figure 11.5).

Each stair represents a linear component, and the spiral structure in which they are embedded represents the cyclic component. In *Leelah*, therapy works by establishing three developmental Sequences for each of the three spirals. The spectrum is structured as a linear oxymoron containing contradictions and paradoxes. In this structure, movement is subjected to the Aristotelian law, which states motion occurs between relevant opposites. When an Avatar is preoccupied with a certain theme, the opposing theme is also necessarily relevant to them, even if it is not tangibly manifest at first (Figure 11.6).

The three Sequences remain the same throughout the therapy. They accompany the Avatar during every session and constitute their key characteristic. The only person consciously aware of them and monitoring them is the therapist. Within each oxymoron, the paradigm defines four types of movement that portray the dialogue between its two poles:

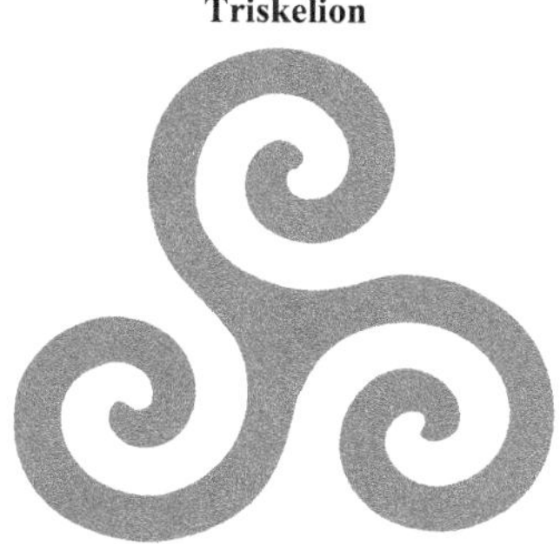

Figure 11.5 Triskelion.

Figure 11.6 Madness sanity.

1 Blocked
2 Sudden
3 Hesitant
4 Harmonic

At the end of each session, the therapist uses these icons to mark the relevant type of movement on individual *Developmental Sequences Tracker* (DST[3]) (See Appendix 1), which is meant for the therapist alone, as she is present in the Transitional Play Space. The therapist's goal is to acquaint each Avatar with all four movement types.

All four movements are equally important for development and are not in any hierarchical relationship with one another. The Sequences are designed to disrupt any oppressive dynamic by which the therapist favours the 'positive' pole over the 'negative' and directs the player towards a particular point on the spectrum. The paradigm wishes to move beyond the linear-hierarchic view and replace it with a circular/spiral one (Blum-Yazdi, 2013). As the ouroboros, accepting them allows both ends of the spectrum to meet, granting it a circular shape. This encounter between opposite poles creates a spinning structure, which sparks yet another revolution of the endless spiral. Illustration of Leelah's Developmental Sequences work is available in the book Behind the Mask, chapter The Leelah Play, Avatar as mask in trauma-informed drama therapy (Blum-Yazdi, 2023).

Summary

The Leelah Play model contains two components. One is the Leelah play paradigm, which is considering three key issues: power relationships, the concept of freedom, and the identity of the playing subject in therapy. The theory embraces a critical outlook on the world of therapy and its possible oppressive dynamics. Therefore, Leelah was created in a manner that is mindful of oppression in therapy and attempts to address it. The principles of this paradigm can be applied in various ways, ranging from verbal conversation to creative arts. The other component of the model, Leelah – Play for Itself, is only one possible application designed to illustrate and demonstrate these principles in action.

The basic assumption of this model is that a group or individual have all the knowledge they need to achieve self-healing. The role of the therapist is to maintain a safe and protected space in which healing can happen while doing her best to avoid any form of intervention. It is the role of the group to bring about healing. This model is suitable for any player with a distinct and stable sense of self and the capacity to engage in Organic Play Space while maintaining their self-identity. The model can be applied partially when working with clients coping with developmental difficulties, mental problems and difficulty discerning the transition between different realities.

In the last 20 years, I have worked through Leelah with ultra-Orthodox men, students, children and youth at risk, people with autism, mental health issues, etc. Throughout those years, I had the good fortune of visiting many therapeutic Leelah towns; and each of these experiences was both profound and wondrous. I am forever grateful to all those devoted players with the lives of whose Avatars I was fortunate enough to interlace the life of my own Avatar for several months. These towns are always with me, treasured in my heart. To my understanding, play for itself has healing potential, and when purpose becomes more important than play, it is not therapy but something else.

To Pazit Ilan-Bercovich and Ornit Horesh, past co-head of the Israeli dramatherapy division, for support, decent collegiality, and professionalism and Salvo Pitruzzella for your friendship, kindness, and love for the text.

Notes

1 The claim of unavoidable intervention origin in Direct/Naive Realism philosophy perception. The claim of unnecessary intervention origin in indirect/representational realism philosophy perception.
2 More details and demos about operating the model are available on site: www.leelahplay.com
3 In the case of a large group, I fulfill a Group DST, and I refer to the group as a whole.

- Both forms are available on site.

References

Axline, V. M. (1964). Nondirective therapy. In M. R. Haworth (Ed), *Child psychotherapy: Practice and theory*. New York: Basic Books, pp. 34–39.

Blum-Yazdi, D. (2013). Language, kwan, world. *Journal of East-West Psychology Quart,* 3(39). Available at: https://www.academia.edu/44315071/Language_Koan_World (Accessed: 1 December 2022).

Blum-Yazdi, D. (2014). Leelah - A play for itself: An undirected model of dramatherapy. In Berger, R. (Ed), *Creation - The therapy heart.* Kiryat Bialik: Ach Books, pp. 67–95.

Blum-Yazdi, D. (2019). *The play paradigm: Theoretical concepts of power, identity and liberty in the therapeutic playing field (doctoral dissertation).* Ramat Gan: Bar Ilan University.

Blum-Yazdi, D. (2023). The Leelah Play, Avatar as mask in trauma-informed drama therapy. In S. Ridley (Ed), *Behind the mask: The expressive use of masks across cultures and healing arts (pending publication)*. London: Routledge.

Capra, F. (2013). The Tao of physics. In M. Cazenave (Ed), *Science and consciousness: Two views of the universe*. Oxford: Pergamon Press, pp. 21–32.

Erikson, E. (1993). *Childhood and society*. New York: W.W. Norton & Company.

Gersie, A. (1987). Dramatherapy and play. In S. Jennings (Ed), *Dramatherapy - theory and practice 1*. London: Routledge, pp. 46–72.

Hougham, R. (2006). Numinosity, symbol and ritual in the Sesame approach. *Dramatherapy*, 28(2), pp. 3–7.

Huizinga, J. (2014). *Homo Ludens: A study of the play-element in culture*. Mansfield: Martino Fine Books.

Husserl, E. (2012). *Ideas: General introduction to pure phenomenology*. Translated from German by W. R. Boyce Gibson. London: Routledge.

Jennings, S. (1995). Playing for real. *International Play Journal*, 3, pp. 132–141.

Jennings, S. (1999). *Introduction to developmental play therapy*. London: Jessica Kingsley

Johnson, D. R. (1992). The drama therapist "in role". In S. Jennings (Ed), *Dramatherapy - theory and practice 2*. London: Routledge, pp. 112–136.

Klein, M. (1959). *The psychoanalysis of children*. London: The Hogarth Press.

Kowalsky, R., Keisari, S., and Raz, N. (2019). Hall of mirrors on stage: An introduction to psychotherapeutic playback theatre. *The Arts in Psychotherapy*, 66, 1–7. 10.1016/j.aip.2019.101577

Lahad, M. (2000). *Creative supervision: The use of expressive arts methods in supervision and self-supervision*. London: Jessica Kingsley.

Landy, R. J. (1996). *Persona and performance: The meaning of role in drama, therapy, and everyday life*. New York: The Guilford Press.

Mook, B. (2003). Phenomenology, analytical psychology, and play therapy. In R. Brooke (Ed), *Pathways into the Jungian world*. London: Routledge, pp. 235–254.

Moreno. J. L. (1944). A case of paranoia treated through psychodrama. *Sociometry*, 7(3), pp. 312–327.

Nietzsche, F. (2001). *Beyond good and evil*. Translated from German by J. Norman. Cambridge: Cambridge University Press.

Pendzik, S. (2006). On dramatic reality and its therapeutic function in drama therapy. *The Arts in Psychotherapy*, 33(4), pp. 271–280.

Pendzik, S. (2008). Dramatic resonances: A technique of intervention in drama therapy, supervision, and training. *The Arts in Psychotherapy*, 35(3), pp. 217–223.

Pitruzzella, S. (2004). *Introduction to dramatherapy: Person and threshold*. Abington: Routledge.

Pitruzzella, S. (2017). *Drama, creativity and intersubjectivity: The roots of change in dramatherapy*. Abington: Routledge.

Rogers, C. R. (2007). *Counseling and psychotherapy*. Boston: Houghton.

Winnicott, D. W. (1975). *Through paediatrics to psychoanalysis: Collected papers*. New York: Basic Books.

Appendix 1 Developmental sequences tracker (DST) - Individual

Developmental Sequences Tracker - INDIVIDUAL

Leelah
Play for Itself

Date: ____________ Mythology Name: ____________

Player Character Name: ____________ Therapist Character Name: ____________

1 D.S. & Transition Types*		Primary Sequence Pole 1 ____ ( ) ____ Pole 2	Secondary Sequence 1 Pole 1 ____ ( ) ____ Pole 2	Secondary Sequence 2 Pole 1 ____ ( ) ____ Pole 2
	ILLUSTRATE			
2 Symptoms & Signs		Symptoms Player ____ Environment ____ Therapist ____	Positive Signs ____ ____ ____ ____	Negative Signs ____ ____ ____ ____
	ILLUSTRATE			
3 Mood & Affect		Player Mood Type ____ Level ____	Player Affect Type ____ Level ____	Correlation: Mood & Affect (×/√) ____
	ILLUSTRATE			
4 Social System		Player Social Status ____	Friends & Opponents ____ | ____ ____ | ____	Connections Quality ____ ____
	ILLUSTRATE			
5 Relationship Therapist & Player		D.S. For Therapist Pole 1 ____ ( ) ____ Pole 2	Support Type Required ____	Relationship Type ____
	ILLUSTRATE			

*Transition Types: 1. Blocked 2. Sudden 3. Hesitant 4. Harmonious

1

2

3

4

5

The table is divided into horizontal rows. There are five sections: (1) Developmental Sequences & Transition Types, (2) Symptoms & Signs, (3) Mood and Affect, (4) Social Status, (5) Relationship with the Therapist. Each section is divided into two rows. The upper rows are for grading the status, and the lower rows explain and illustrate actions, behaviour, or events portrayed during play.

Note

A mythology name is a short descriptive name made up of a few words describing the character. Examples: 'Deep Roots,' 'Dancing Flame,' and 'Sphinx.'

Index

Note: Italic page numbers refer to figures and "n" indicates endnote in the text.

For Product Safety Concerns and Information please contact our EU representative GPSR@taylorandfrancis.com
Taylor & Francis Verlag GmbH, Kaufingerstraße 24, 80331 München, Germany

www.ingramcontent.com/pod-product-compliance
Lightning Source LLC
Chambersburg PA
CBHW060258220326
41598CB00027B/4155

* 9 7 8 1 0 3 2 2 0 8 7 4 9 *